SEARCHING FOR THE STORK

SEARCHING FOR THE STORK

by
Marion Lee Wasserman

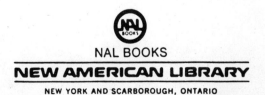

NAL BOOKS

NEW AMERICAN LIBRARY

NEW YORK AND SCARBOROUGH, ONTARIO

Published simultaneously in Canada by The New American Library of Canada Limited

NAL TRADEMARK REG. U.S. PAT. OFF. AND FOREIGN COUNTRIES
REGISTERED TRADEMARK—MARCA REGISTRADA
HECHO EN CHICAGO, U.S.A.

SIGNET, SIGNET CLASSIC, MENTOR, ONYX, PLUME, MERIDIAN
and NAL BOOKS are published *in the United States* by NAL
PENGUIN INC., 1633 Broadway, New York, New York 10019,
in Canada by The New American Library of Canada Limited,
81 Mack Avenue, Scarborough, Ontario M1L 1M8

Library of Congress Cataloging-in-Publication Data

Wasserman, Marion Lee.
  Searching for the stork.

  1. Wasserman, Marion Lee—Health.   2. Pregnancy,
Complications of—Patients—United States—Biography.
3. Pregnancy, Complications of—Psychological aspects.
4. Childlessness—Psychological aspects.   I. Title.
RG571.W37A3 1988   618.3 [B]   87-28221
ISBN 0-453-00594-2

Designed by Sherry Brown

First Printing, May, 1988

1 2 3 4 5 6 7 8 9

PRINTED IN THE UNITED STATES OF AMERICA

for Dean,
with love and gratitude

ACKNOWLEDGMENTS

For their friendship, encouragement and wise advice, I thank my early readers, Elaine de Mers, Allan Keiler, Lynn Klamkin, Howard Norman and Jane Shore.

I am also deeply grateful to my editor, Alexia Dorszynski, and my agent, Meredith Bernstein.

Finally, my thanks to Dean. In addition to the other roles he has played in my life, he has been an invaluable editor of this book, incisive and supportive from first to last. He never begrudged me his time or judgment, and whenever my faith in this project flagged, his was there, carrying me forward.

In telling my story, I have changed some minor details and the names of many of the people mentioned; other than that, this is a true story.

What could be more moving, significant or true: every force and hidden chance in the universe has so combined that a certain thing was the way it was.
—James Agee, *Let Us Now Praise Famous Men*

SEARCHING FOR THE STORK

A LETTER

April 1984

Dear Amelia,

For me, you existed, you were. Should I say you lived?
You did, and you didn't.

I saw you move. There you were! There was your image
computerized into two dimensions, presented to me on a
screen as though you were an astronaut floating somewhere
thousands of miles away. How strange it was, lying on an
examining table in theaterlike darkness, looking into your
world, my inner space. Your slightest motion—so independent!
—seemed the beginning of all beginnings, a primal experiment.
The first time I saw you, you brought your stub-fingered
hand to your mouth in seeming anticipation of having a thumb
to suck. And another day your rabbitlike legs suddenly stretched
out and up, as though you had somewhere to go and your
floating could float you through rooms.

You were never interchangeable with anyone, never replaceable.
Yet I knew so little about you.

I thought of you all the time. Chose my food with you in
mind; made extra sure not to fall or get hit because you might
be hurt; pressed my hands against my belly, which was as
close as I could come to touching you . . . until the end. And
you were the greater treasure for your hiddenness and
secretness. Your emergence would be a miracle, a blooming,

that would, I had every reason to hope, last my lifetime and continue beyond it.

How can I not wonder if in any sense you knew yourself? Why should I deny it? You seemed so peaceful, flexing and floating there in your black, soft world. I keep wondering, did you know peace? Did you know pain and fear, as I did, when the time came, too early, for you to leave your drifting? Did you know love, sense it somehow in our connectedness, our shared substance and form?

Soon it will be the first anniversary of your death. (Death? What a queer word for one who never lived outside the womb, never felt the world's assaultive greeting.) How fast the months have gone by, how automatically you tumble into the past.

I find myself wondering, for the first time since you died, whether Dean and I should have accepted your ashes and scattered them in some quiet place where we could have gone now to be near you. Perhaps. But I console myself with the thought that I have a place to seek your presence in: the home of all your days and nights, as constant, sturdy and dependable a shell as ever housed a snail. My sweet mollusk, my soft one, what place could be more yours than this vessel you left behind?

CHAPTER 1

FANTASY

1

At the age of twenty-three, thirteen years before I wrote that letter to Amelia, I went to a funeral for the first time in my life—the funeral of a little boy four years old. I was married then but not to Dean. My husband sang at the funeral service, and behind him on a raised platform before the room of mourners was a pale blue coffin; the color and the shortness of it gave it a sinister fascination.

"We're glad Andrew was born. At least we had these four years with him." I kept hearing in my mind what my friend had said when she called to tell me her son was dead. I was like a faithless stranger witnessing through a sanctuary window the liturgy of the faithful. The quality of my friend's love humbled and mystified me. In those days I could only wonder, how could parenthood be worth so much, worth even an agony of grief? I couldn't understand it. I felt lucky to be childless.

My first marriage lasted eight and a half years, and not once did my husband and I try to conceive a child. Whenever one of us suggested that now, maybe now, would be a good time, the other one pointed out the

1

reasons for waiting, and the suggestion, tentative at best, was withdrawn.

After we got divorced, I wondered if I had squandered the only chance I would ever have to become a mother. Yet I was grateful not to have a mother's responsibilities and not to be fighting over custody and visitation. Grateful that my husband and I had been so hesitant, sensing all along that having a child would not be right. In truth, I had never really wanted to create a person half me, half him. I had always been secretly afraid of duplicating the tame little boy of his childhood snapshots.

Yet I used to wonder if something was wrong with me. Why didn't I feel pressed to be a mother, like so many of my friends, whose longing for children was aggressive, incautious? Why were my other urges paramount—to learn, to travel, to work, to be alone? Was I unfeminine? Would I ever change? Why did the emotional hazards of motherhood and the physical hazards of pregnancy and delivery so frighten me? I could see that most of my friends who had children were no better adjusted, no more capable, than I, and some had even more troubled marriages.

In those days, whenever a friend had a baby I was one of the first visitors, lured to the spectacle of a newborn child. Every hospital had the same wide window with a lineup of infants sleeping or bawling on the other side of the glass in dishpan-sized beds of clear plastic. I remember one friend I went to visit had her baby daughter in her room with her, nursing. I wasn't permitted to enter with the baby there, so I just stood awhile at the door, watching. The baby's face was red, working against the cushion of flesh.

I loved buying presents for my friends' babies. Part of the fun of a birth was the excuse it gave me to pick my way through displays of bibs and rattles and soft toys, miniature shirts and pants and dresses. For one friend's newborn girl I bought an embroidered pinafored dress she would outgrow in a few months.

I was twenty-six and in the sixth year of my first marriage when I noticed something I had never noticed before, something as familiar to me as my own breathing: a fantasy child, a daughter in my own image. An inquisitive little girl; pretty, with wavy dark brown hair and anxious green eyes. I had been tutoring her in the puzzles and pleasures of life for so many years that I couldn't say when she had been born. I spoke to her at moments of discovery or reflection. Anything that might make her life happy was worth imparting, however trivial. She listened attentively to everything I told her, especially to the lessons revealed by my mistakes.

When I first noticed my child's Pucklike appearances, I had the same surprised sensation as when I once read a description of dust drifting in a sunbeam. How could it be that I had delighted in those shifting, glistening motes as a child lying in bed mornings and yet never noticed my noticing? Like the mote-filled beam, the daughter of my mental dialogues was so elementary I hadn't given her any thought.

Now I thought more and more about what she meant: I did, after all, have a desire to be a mother. It was a fundamental desire, easily ignored, easily denied, even as it molded my daydreams.

At about this time, my husband told me about a woman he had talked to at one of his professional conferences. Married, childless, in her late forties, she told him she had never wanted a child until it was too late, when she began longing to have one. That woman scared him, and she scared me.

Out of fear, not longing, I suggested to my husband that we get started. He rejected the idea, and about two years later we were divorced. The specter of the childless forty-year-old stood before me with a new vividness.

2

I was thirty-four when I conceived Amelia. I had never conceived a child before. It was January 12, 1983. I'm sure of the date (as sure as one can be) because I'd been keeping a chart of my temperature for two months, wanting to determine whether I was ovulating (what if I'm not normal, I kept thinking) and wanting to help things along all I could. The way I saw it, there I was on the carousel, and there, streaking by, was the gold ring. Each year I would whirl towards it twelve times. That didn't sound like many chances, really—not at my age.

I put the thermometer in my mouth at six A.M. and dozed off, holding my head still, making a fish face to keep the cold glass in place under my tongue. Then, waking, trying to get more comfortable, I replaced the thermometer in its box on my night table and went back to sleep. Later I saw that my temperature was down to 97.1.

I called Dean at work. "Can you possibly get home early?" He was a lawyer, commuting to Boston each day from our house in the suburbs, working long hours in the corporate department of a large law firm. I was practicing law in Boston then too, but only half-time, and half-heartedly. I worked on sundry matters in a smoky four-lawyer office on Beacon Street near the State House. Often I thought of the job I had had during my first marriage, teaching writing to college students, and I missed it. Law school, I sometimes thought, had been a mistake for me. But then I remembered that it couldn't have been a mistake. Dean and I had met there. Registration day. September 8, 1976. Nine, eight, seven, six. He had followed me into the bookstore.

"This may sound silly," I said now, "but I think we should have sex before dinner. I've ovulated, I'm almost positive."

He laughed. "I suspect that an hour one way or the other isn't going to make much difference. You know, this isn't such a precise . . ."

"Yeah, maybe so, but this is the first month the drop in temperature has been so obvious. It's our best chance yet, I really think so." Inside me was this microscopic speck of an egg that according to the books would only last about twenty-four hours and might already be near extinction.

"Look, I'll do my best to get the early train, but don't worry so much. We'll get you knocked up, if not this month, next month."

After we made love, I drew a circle around the dot on my temperature chart. There were other circles for that week, but this was the only one hanging so far down. By the next day (my temperature had climbed to 97.85) it looked like the tip of an icicle. That point marked the fourteenth day of my cycle. By day thirty-five, my temperature was above 98 and still rising (though slightly now) and my period hadn't started.

I compared my chart repeatedly with the one I had photocopied from a library book on fertility. Could this be it, I kept thinking. Could we be so fortunate—after only three months of trying? What would it be like? This reaching toward doubleness, it was so new, I might have been trying to slip unharmed through a sheet of glass, or to travel inside my body to find there the center of the earth. This was magic: distracting, exciting, unnerving. I called my health center and heard the nurse saying, "Yes, it does sound like you're pregnant."

There had been a time when I wasn't sure Dean would ever want a child. "I can't deal with that now,"

he said a few days after we decided to get married. He was standing in the kitchen of our apartment, his weight shifted forward to his right leg, like a warning. He ran his long fingers through his fine wheat-colored hair, pulling it back, away from his forehead, the way he has a habit of doing when his hair gets too long. "One thing at a time. That issue isn't real to me yet. I may not want children, I don't know." I felt empty inside when he said that, as though my body was one of those outlines the police draw on the ground at the scene of a crime. I was afraid I would faint. What would life be like if I were never to become a mother, not by my choice, but by Dean's? What would happen to our marriage?

"Don't you have a fantasy child?" I asked, sitting down at the table to steady myself. "You know, a kid you chat with in your imagination? A little boy you teach things to?" I looked up at Dean. He was leaning on the kitchen counter; not against it, but on it. He was tall enough—over six feet—to spread his hand flat on the counter and lean his weight into it.

"No, I don't."

I had assumed everyone had such a child; without that mental tug toward parenthood, Dean might never come around.

How much did he count in my life, how much did I love him, as against this child I was daydreaming about?

When I married him a few months later, I was sure of my choice. I loved him more than my imagined child; and I believed that if we loved each other enough we would find answers. An ingenuous faith perhaps, but simple and reassuring and in retrospect wise.

For a year or so, we stayed off the subject of having children. Newly married, moving out of our apartment into a house, there was excitement enough in our lives without thinking about having kids. But one day I broke the taboo. All of a sudden I was peeved. If Dean thought he could wait several years and then opt for fatherhood, he wasn't being fair. Hadn't he read any of those articles about the risks for older women? How old would I be by the time we talked about it? Thirty-five? Forty?

"How about fifty?" That was Dean. Always getting a laugh out of me. Even when I was angry.

"Let me cogitate on it." That was Dean too. Always "cogitating" when I was impatient to decide something.

Then one Saturday morning in bed, "Let's not bother with that," he said when I reached toward my night table for my diaphragm.

"What?" Suddenly I was the one unready to change the status quo. "Do you think we should? Aren't you scared?"

"Of course I'm scared."

Afterwards (we were hugging each other, giggling, nervous, with sperm leaking out of me, wetting my buttocks, wetting the sheet) I had a sense of the space inside me: space just waiting, set, for something magic to take place, to proceed in the dark all on its own without help, without guidance. So different, so different this was, from any time before.

3

The nurse's hunch was just that, after all, like mine. I had yet to have a test—*the* test—the traditional verdict. I had yet to hear the absolute pronouncement: "Marion, you're pregnant." I had to restrain my giddy readiness to celebrate.

"The routine test is a urine test," the nurse explained to me over the phone. She had an accent that sounded Jamaican, and an oddly muffled voice, as though she had a wad of cotton in her mouth. "It's not likely to give a positive result for at least another week, six weeks from the start of your last period." Damn, I thought, another week.

"No," she said, "they don't use rabbits anymore. No animals."

I woke Dean out of a purring sleep the night before the test. He whimpered and hugged his shoulders. It was three A.M. "I couldn't hold it in," I whispered. "The urine sample, do you think it needs to be refrigerated?"

The nurse had instructed me not to eat or drink anything after midnight and to collect the urine first thing in the morning. From this I reasoned that the first specimen after midnight was the one the lab would need.

Dean half-raised his eyelids and looked at me. "Huh?" I repeated my question.

"Refrigerated? I never heard of putting urine in the refrigerator." He closed his eyes and turned away, tugging the covers to his chin. "I'm cold."

Though I had a nagging recollection of refrigerating urine at some doctor's instructions years before, I left the jar of urine under the bathroom sink. This was a scientific matter, and Dean was savvy in such things. "Mr. Wizard," I often called him. He had been a chemistry major in college and had taught high school physics for a year. He almost always had answers for my questions—answers I tended to forget. It was the questions that stayed in my mind. Why does fog form over snowy fields? Why does salt melt snow? Things like that.

The next morning, the receptionist at the lab had me go into the bathroom to pour my urine from the Sweet Life jam jar into a plastic cup labeled with my name and health plan number. When I returned to her with the cup, it occurred to me to mention the problem of the night before.

"Oh dear," she said, looking up at me, her eyes level

with the countertop and the cup of golden liquid. "You should have put it in the refrigerator. There's really no point in having this analyzed."

I was surprised to feel tears coming into my eyes. "Are you absolutely sure? I just went to the bathroom, so I can't possibly give you a new specimen." The woman disappeared through the doorway of an office adjoining the reception area. When she came back, she handed me an empty plastic cup.

"Try. My supervisor says we don't need much, but it has to be fresh."

Returning from the bathroom, I held up a cup containing barely a teaspoon of urine. "I don't know if they can work with this little," the woman said. She disappeared again into the back room, taking the cup with her, then reemerged and placed it on a metal cart neatly crowded with specimens of blood and urine. "Maybe they can get a result with this, maybe not. Anyhow, if not, you'll have to come back Monday. The lab is closed over the weekend. Call your doctor after four today."

I went to the pay phone in the stairwell and called Dean at his office. "I don't think we're going to find out anything today. The urine wasn't any good. It did need to be in the refrig, like I thought." I was surprised how upset and angry I sounded.

"Hey, Frog, c'mon," Dean said, using the nickname he had pulled out of the air years ago. I was almost always Frog or Froggie or Froggo between the two of us, almost never Marion. "The weekend's not such a long time. And you don't even have to go back on Monday. I'll drop your sample off for you on my way to work. I'm sorry I was wrong." My spitefulness dissolved. After all, Dean was feeling the disappointment too.

At four, I called the obstetrics nurse again, the one with the Jamaican accent and the cottony voice. "Congratulations!" she said, "You're pregnant!"

"I am? I am?"

*   *   *

Soon after my pregnancy test I began feeling the oppressive fatigue that was to last until early April. The nurse assured me that my complaint was characteristic of the first trimester.

On a February visit with friends in Vermont, I spent most of the weekend on the couch, dozing or reading. Everyone moved around me, catering to my wishes, making an excited fuss over my being pregnant. On Sunday morning, while Dean went with our friends and two other guests to hike in the snow, I lay inside wondering what the guests, who didn't know me, must think of me. Even allowing for my being pregnant, how unlikably leaden and self-absorbed I must seem.

I got up and put on my hiking boots and my jacket and followed the others outside. My legs resisted motion; I had to consider each step I took in the heavy boots, even when I stayed out of the ankle-deep snow and kept to the plowed road. Trudging up the steep rise in the road to see where the others had gone, I gulped the cold air like a tonic after being inside near the fire. The sound of my hard breathing moved with me. From a point partway up the incline, I could see Dean and the others working their separate zigzagging paths through the dense, leafless brush on the hillside, their figures brightly colored against the white slope, progressing slowly as spiders toward the long ridge at the top. Their effort seemed herculean to me. I lay down on the crusty snow, spread-eagle, arms out, and stared into the blue of the sky, marveling at my inability to act the tomboy as I loved to do, telling myself to enjoy the change. There was something luxurious in having a socially acceptable excuse for such lassitude, an excuse not linked to illness, an excuse enviable, chosen: creation. I moved my legs and arms in the snow, like kids do, making an angel. The cold soaked through my long johns and blue jeans, but I lay there, fingering a stalk of dried grass that poked through the snow, until I heard Dean's deep voice (that I had listened to and held to, as though reeling him towards me, closer and closer) parting the air above me, soothing and attentive. "Help you up, Froggo?"

4

From the beginning, I scrutinized my flat-bellied, small-breasted body for signs of change. My breasts were slightly fuller than usual, but they were like that most months for the four or five days ending one menstrual cycle and beginning the next, so this was nothing astonishing. By late February, my abdomen was beginning to swell—but slowly, ever so slowly. The slight tightness in the waistline of my skirts and slacks told me more than my image in the mirror.

A friend of Dean's loaned us *A Child is Born*, a book of photographs of life within the womb. Now I could see what was happening inside me. The embryo, floating in a transparent, baggy sac, was an otherworldly creature, itself transparent, so the red of the veins and arteries and liver and heart could be seen through the colorless skin. The oversized, cretinous-looking head had lidless eyes, dark pools, darkest at the edges, as big as the already visible crescents of the ears. "Six weeks from conception, one-half inch," the caption read. "The baby is growing. With rapid beats the heart pumps the blood from its small circulatory system out into the immense tree of vessels in the placenta, where millions of villi absorb nourishment and oxygen for the little body."

On March 16, I hear it myself, insisting that it is there inside me, it is real. I have two hearts!

The nurse uses an odd-looking stethoscope, pressing the flat, blunt end of it, shaped like the head of an electric razor, against my lower abdomen, just above the line of my pubic hair, where she first coats my skin with a grayish gel. I'm tense waiting for her to find the sound. "Sometimes we can't hear it at eleven weeks," she says. "That's perfectly normal." Normal or not, I know I'll worry if she has to give up. I'm not even thinking about my getting to hear the heart, just worrying about everything being all right. "There it is," the nurse says suddenly, and she puts the plugs in my ears. The beating is vigorous and regular; a thick sound, but mysteriously rapid, the way I imagine the heartbeat of a small, nervous creature—a rabbit, or a mouse. I'm so astounded, I can't look at the nurse. If I had my own stethoscope, I would listen to that beating for hours.

At eleven weeks, my abdomen had a new roundness, a shape I associated with other women, not with me. I wondered if I would ever again be flat across the stomach. My waistline was disappearing, too, the indentation above each hip filling in, so that I had more and more the shape of an upright dog. Unable any longer to quite zip up the suit skirts I wore to work or to close the fly on my jeans, I went shopping for maternity clothes.

By April first, my belly had expanded higher up, under my ribs, and was noticeably rounder at the sides. I looked down at it, rested my hands on it—a little dome, a little house, for my fetus-child. I could no longer wear my skirts, even with the zippers slightly open, so I began wearing my maternity clothes, enjoying the public declaration they made.

I was an eager pupil. Even before the nurse began talking, I was thumbing through the folder of printed material: "Your Prenatal Diet," "Prenatal Exercises," "Sex During Pregnancy." At the top of the page about sex, the male and female scientific symbols interlocked circles, and a baby in a fetal position slept upside down inside the circle of the female sign. Did they really hug themselves so tightly, tuck themselves into such a compact bundle? With my pen, I traced the curve of the skull and spine and buttocks.

There were six other women in the nutrition class at my health center, all of them, like me, about to enter the second trimester of pregnancy. Two of them raised their hands when the nurse asked if any of us had children. I was glad not to know whatever it was they knew. I enjoyed thinking of myself as "having my first." But the two mothers had my admiration—they were seasoned graduates hoping for a few pointers; I was a novice, a simpleton.

The nurse held up a chart, and I dutifully pulled one like it from my folder—color photographs of food grouped into columns labeled *Milk, Meat, Fruit-Vegetable, Grain, Other*. The nurse laid a plastic lamb chop, a plastic wedge of cheese, and some plastic vegetables on the table in front of her as she talked about serving sizes and the nutritional requirements of fetuses and pregnant women. I looked over my chart, happy as any first-grader to rest my eyes on the pictures: a watermelon slice, a chocolate pudding, a tuna fish salad.

After the class, I got in line at the pharmacy behind one of the two mothers. She stepped away each time a little blond boy disappeared behind a wall or chair or person. "Brian!" She pulled him into line with her, but he was off again, tottering towards some object of curiosity—a table littered with magazines; a purse set down by an unsuspecting patient; another little child, tottering like himself. Finally, his mother reached the counter and handed her prescription through the window. Then it was my turn. "Prenatal vitamins." A shibboleth. I said it with the pride of the initiate as I pushed the prescription across the counter. The vitamins were capsules, bright blue, not tablets as I had expected, and the flat-sided white bottle held enough of them for three months. I would need to be sure to keep to a schedule, every morning or every evening; "best taken after meals," the nurse had said. I liked the jiggle of the capsules inside the bottle, and the odd, Swedish-sounding brand name: Pampren Forte.

I Scotch-taped my food chart to the inside of a cupboard door at home. The photographs of food had a reassuring simplicity, like the blue vitamins. For the next week, I was obsessed with serving sizes and food groups, and I put more meat on my plate at lunch and dinner than I liked to have. My appetite diminished, and I threw out most of the meat. "Forget the chart," Dean told me. "Just put it away, you'll do fine without it." I was relieved to follow his advice, but I still kept drinking extra milk, twice as much as I was used to, buying milk now in gallons instead of half-gallons. The gallon container in the refrigerator was an unfamiliar sight I associated with large families. It was one of the odd transformations that sometimes made me edgy. Added expense, less room, heavier load; it was beginning already, months before the birth.

On the train, going to work, I read the *Complete Guide to Breastfeeding* (embarrassed, covering the title and pictures with my hands). At home, I read the *Jane Fonda Workout Book for Pregnancy, Birth, and Recovery*, a gift Dean had given me when my pregnancy test came out positive. Both books helped me teach myself what to anticipate from my body and how to care for it and the creature inside.

The more I read about breastfeeding, the more I envisioned myself feeding my newborn my own milk. How beautiful we would be together! "The nursing couple," the book called us. I didn't want Dean to be shut out of the feeding process, though. Perhaps we could each handle half of the feedings—me with my breasts, Dean with bottles. The nurse said that wasn't unusual.

"Oh, boring!" was my mother's response over the phone when I told her my plan to nurse.

"Boring?"

"Oh, yes. You'll be so bored with it."

"You didn't nurse, did you?"

"No, I never wanted to. It's very uncomfortable, a real nuisance. And babies bite. Grandma got bitten so badly with Uncle Ansel her nipples got infected."

"Well, this book I'm reading talks about biting; it can be prevented."

"Not with some babies it can't."

"Well, it's really healthier for a baby to have mother's milk than formula. There's a reason nature provides a mother with milk."

"You and Steve were never deprived because you were on formula."

"I didn't say a baby can't do well on formula. It's just that, all things considered, mother's milk is the best way."

"You'll change your mind." My mother's voice was high and rising on the word "you'll."

I tried to chuckle indifferently. "How's the weather out there? Is the snow all gone?"

The Jane Fonda workout book had nothing to do with Jane Fonda except that it had a cover photo of her in a black leotard posing with the book's author and two other women, one of whom held an infant and one of whom was pregnant, and it had a foreword by Fonda explaining her personal connection with the author and talking about her childbearing. There were also several black and white photos of Fonda and her infant son, including one of her nursing. Dean took a critical interest in that photo, staring at it for a while, handing the book back to me, then insisting, "Let me see that again." I laughed. "Trying to form an opinion about nursing, huh?" Dean's lust for Fonda was a long-standing joke between us.

The so-called "pregnancy workout" was strenuous,

and the book convinced me of the need to be in good physical condition for the ordeal of giving birth. I added the lengthy exercise routine to the daily yoga routine I already maintained (or tried to maintain). The book's inclusion of a "recovery workout" went at least a small way towards easing my fears about getting back into shape after the birth. I didn't need to read it yet, but it was there, an insurance policy.

Some of the book's bizarre dos and don'ts warned me that my caring for myself might sometimes conflict with my caring for the baby inside me. The baby, of course, would have to rule. Prolonged hot baths, for example, were dangerous, raising body temperature enough after fifteen minutes or so to damage the fetal nervous system. Doing strenuous exercise while lying down on my back could also be a problem. The weight of my uterus pressing on the vein pumping blood to my heart could hinder my circulation and the baby's. "Don't worry, do your exercises," the nurse said when I asked her about this. "When you get very big, it'll start to bother you. You'll know when to quit, but it won't be for quite a while, maybe your thirtieth week." I was terrified of harming the baby.

The workout book also had a chapter on "Preparing for Labor and Birth." When the time came, in my seventh month, for the childbirth classes at the health center, Dean and I could read this chapter together. There was no point trying to absorb all this scary advice yet, about contractions and pushing and breathing, about how important it would be to be prepared, me for the physical struggle, Dean for the role of "coach." There was still plenty of time to get to all that (though the weeks did slip by with unsettling speed).

There was one chapter of the book I avoided reading: "Dealing with Problems and Complications." I had no way of knowing that one small section of this chapter, three brief, sensitively written paragraphs, would soon be the only part of the book I would want to look at. It was called "Handling Grief." It started: "It happens rarely now, but still an infant occasionally does not survive."

I had faith that sometime within a week or two of my due date, October 7, I would give birth to an infant and that infant would survive. I must have had faith, because I permitted myself feelings of joyous expectation and in many ways acted as though my child's arrival was a certainty. I bought a sock monkey—the startled-looking kind I had always wanted as a kid, with a brown and white knit body and wide, bright red lips, and a long tail sewn to a red sock-heel rump—and I put it in the room Dean and I were going to fix up for the baby. I brought home complimentary copies of baby magazines from the maternity shops and read all the articles about newborns and set them aside to refer to after I gave birth. I told people, "Dean and I are going to be parents in October."

As my belly expanded, I thought it looked asymmetrical—more swollen on the right side than on the left. I asked Dean what he thought. Yes, he saw the asymmetry, too. We told ourselves it must be perfectly ordinary, or perhaps it was caused by my scoliotic spine—my right and left sides have always been misaligned, and my right hip is higher than my left.

In mid-April I had my first meeting with Dr. Barrie, the obstetrician my health center assigned to me. She saw the asymmetry, too, but she had only two possible explanations for it: either I was carrying twins, or I had a fibroid tumor in my abdomen. The likely explanation was the second one.

I felt suddenly weak, like a rag doll, and I was glad I was sitting down. Dr. Barrie said the tumor, assuming I had one, probably wouldn't be harmful to my pregnancy, but she added that sometimes fibroids grow as large as watermelons and begin competing with the fetus for nourishment. When that happens, the mother has to be hospitalized. The doctor's voice kept on, calm, adult to adult, and I struggled to hear it, wanting only to curl up on the floor like a child. Fibroids, she explained, are benign tumors that feed on the increased supply of blood and estrogen during pregnancy. They often shrink when the pregnancy is over, eliminating the need for an operation.

Things weren't going according to the books—not the books I had at home. Dr. Barrie pointed to pictures of fibroids in her medical text, trying to help me and Dean understand. To me, the illustrations looked hideous. I was revolted by the thought of this round mass (the size of an orange, the doctor said it must be) inside me where the baby was.

On the afternoon of April 20, Dean met me at the radiologist's office in Cambridge where I was scheduled to have a sonogram to determine for certain what the swelling was. I didn't know it then, but that sonogram was to be the first of many—like a dream repeating itself with sinister variations.

That day, at least, the bad news was not a surprise: I did indeed have a fibroid tumor the size of an orange. But there was good news, too. The baby was doing well.

I lay on the table in the semidarkness, my belly smeared with translucent gel. The doctor pressed hard against my abdomen with a sensor like the one the nurse had used to hear the heartbeat. The mottled black and white and gray streaks within the wedge-shaped field on the screen shifted like clouds, and at the center of the wedge a profiled skull and stunted arm and rabbit leg appeared and disappeared, frustratingly vague, yet unquestionably, eerily human, and less than human, like all those pictures in the book at home. I was hypnotized, awed.

Dr. Abram leaned over the table, a large-featured, bosomy redhead wearing a black skirt and tight black

sweater, looking, as Dean said later, like a cross between an earth mother and a she-devil. I flinched as
she pressed into me. "It hurts."

"It shouldn't hurt." She continued to probe, watching the screen. "The fetus looks good. See the pulse
there?" She pointed to a faint throbbing. "That's the
heart beating."

Each time she found an image that interested her,
she pressed a button and a camera clicked somewhere
inside the machine. She was quick; not a word or move
wasted. In four or five minutes, she was finished. She
handed me a towel to wipe the jelly off my abdomen,
and she handed Dean a photograph. Her voice was
deep, loud for the small room, jarring against the mys-
tery. "Here's your first baby picture."

5

I think it was Dean who made up the name—it
sounds like one of his inventions. At any rate, early in
my pregnancy we began referring to "Johnny-Judy."

"Johnny-Judy is hungry," I would tell Dean, looking
down at my belly. "Maybe we should get some lobster."

Or as Dean and I rushed across the commuter parking lot to catch the morning train: "Wait," I would say,
"Johnny-Judy and I can't run that fast."

We never used the name in front of anyone else, but
between the two of us we needed a label other than
"the baby" or "it." "Johnny-Judy" gave us a working
name—a way of speaking about the present and practicing for the future. (Dean, at the opening of baseball
season: "I hope Johnny-Judy will like the Red Sox more
than you do." Me, imagining Dean steering a kid
through the Fenway turnstile: "I hope so too. I can stay
home then without feeling guilty.")

When I speculated about who Johnny-Judy would turn out to be, I felt powerless. Sometimes frightened. One of my worst fears was simply that my child would be unlikable—a jerk. Because there were so few details within my control, or Dean's, those that were became subjects of passionate debate, as we each experimented with our private visions, feeling now close to the child, now estranged, now satisfied, now disappointed.

"If it's a boy, he's got to be circumcised," I insisted. Dean had read *The Circumcision Decision*, a pamphlet distributed by our health center, and it had persuaded him that circumcision was medically unnecessary. "If it ain't broke, don't fix it," he said. But my mind was closed. Circumcision was necessary to mark my child as part of my world—the world of my religion, the world of my lovemaking. How could a Jewish mother have a little boy who wasn't circumcised? And wouldn't such a child seem foreign, or even repulsive, to me? I had never even seen an uncircumcised man.

"You're being awfully stubborn," Dean said. "Why do you want to cut off part of the kid's dick for nothing?"

"You're angry with me, aren't you?"

"Well, I wish you'd at least consider the arguments on the other side."

"Oh well, it may not even be a boy." That ended the conversation, but Dean and I knew we ought to resolve the issue before our baby was born. I put the subject out of my mind for a while on the assumption that if we had a boy Dean would agree to his being circumcised, if only to avoid my sullenness. As it turned out, we never discussed circumcision again. Arguing over it had been a luxury.

Naming was another choice which Dean and I could make—indeed, would have to make—about our child's identity. We lay in bed at night before shutting off the lights and paged through our three-by-three-inch Dell book of baby names, entertaining each other with suggestions. Dean had his refrain: "I still think it should be Ira Reilly if it's a boy, Delilah Reilly if it's a girl."

After a few weeks we had rejected between us almost every name in the book, but then, with a fervor that took us both by surprise, we each began promoting one or two favorites.

We finally settled on a thoroughly Irish name for a boy: Brendan Francis Reilly. I liked the sound of it, the rhythm. I even liked tripping the r's a little, putting on an Irish brogue. What a name for a writer! I had to remind myself that Brendan might have no interest in writing. I hoped at least he would appreciate his name.

I wondered if Brendan Francis Reilly would mind the Francis, would think it odd or sissy. I convinced myself he would like having the same middle name as Dean and his father, and would like having a name chosen to honor Dean's grandfather, Frank Reilly, who had recently died at the age of ninety-five. The Jewish tradition of naming a child after a deceased loved one was, I thought, a comforting one for the child as well as the parents.

I hadn't known Frank Reilly any better than Brendan would, had never met him, but I was willing to subscribe to Dean's portrait of a likable man. I wanted to believe that Frank Reilly, father of Alphonse Francis and grandfather of Dean Francis, had been good-humored like his offspring. I wanted to believe that Dean's unquarrelsome relation with life was an inherited capacity. Brendan, I thought, will be like his father.

Dean and I had more trouble agreeing on a name for a girl. I made my choice quickly and then pressured Dean to accept it. Not wanting to be coerced, and not immediately attracted to the name I had chosen, Dean insisted that I consider other names, Jennifer and Lisa, for example, names he preferred. I tried to think well of his candidates, but I couldn't. There was only one name I wanted for my daughter—the given name of my maternal grandmother whom I had known as Grandma Mollie but whose real name I had discovered on her marriage license after her death. It was, I thought, prettier than Mollie: Amelia. Why my grandmother had changed it I didn't know, but I would bring it back, connecting my daughter to my grandmother's love, a love I had felt to be unwavering.

I was exuberant when Dean one day surprised me by announcing that Amelia would be our daughter's name. How tantalizing my fancied daughter became then. She had a name! Irrepressibly now, I began hoping and hoping for a little girl.

The last week in April, Dean and I went to Florida. The weather was the quintessence of spring—sunny days warm enough for wearing shorts; clear, sweater-cool evenings. All winter I had been planning this trip, a family reunion of sorts for me, and a chance to introduce Dean to my brother and to other relatives he hadn't met. My family, extending to cousins and second cousins, swarmed like bees in a way I remembered from childhood when I lived in Queens, when none of my relatives had to come from any farther than Brooklyn or Long Island to visit. There were twelve of us around the dinner table the first night at my Aunt Louise's, and Dean was abashed but a good sport.

My aunts and sister-in-law exclaimed over how big my belly was, and everyone, it seemed to me, greeted me with special enthusiasm. I took my aunts aside and showed them the photograph of the fetus.

As the week progressed, my aunts were flatteringly amused by the extent of my wardrobe. "Another outfit! Look at her, how pretty!" When I sat down, my clothes lay upon me caressingly—the soft cloth of the purple dress stippled with tiny white and blue flowers; the white blouse with puffy sleeves and lacy yoke my mother had sent me. My billowy clothes got fuller and fuller of me as the days passed. There was one dress I hadn't brought on the trip; it was too big to look right on me yet, but it would be something new to wear in my third trimester.

*   *   *

At Disney World—children everywhere, babies toddling, babies in strollers—look at me, I kept thinking, look at Dean. There are three of us! The kiddie rides, the balloons, the ice cream smeared mouths, the parents lifting their children to their shoulders to view the parade—it was like seeing a movie of a country we were planning to move to, forever. I wanted the people there to know we were coming.

But sometimes I wished I wasn't pregnant, even though I wanted a child; sometimes I resented the way the fetus inside me controlled my life. The biggest rides at Disney World—the kind of amusement park rides I loved but hadn't had a chance to go on in years—were open to Dean but not to me. A sign by the entrance to Space Mountain advised pregnant women to stay off, and when I got in line at Thunder Mountain I was swiftly approached by a security guard who drawled, "Excuse me, ma'am, are you expectin'?" While Dean went on the rides without me, I sulked like a sick child excluded from a game. Sitting on a stone ledge along one of the rosebeds, I stared angrily at my belly, letting my eyes fill with tears, and when Dean came back to me I cried and refused at first to be consoled.

My pregnancy was a physical handicap. When I was least concerned about it, someone else told me I ought to be, and when no one else seemed to notice it, I was frightened and protective.

I had always liked the fake scares of a haunted house, but in the Haunted House at Disney World the crowd shoving in the dark was a genuine menace to me and my child. My hands jumped to my belly, hugging it, and I yelled at a boy who pushed me, and I grabbed Dean's hand and pressed against his back. "Stay in front of me." I could almost feel what it would be like if there were real bats in the air, the fur of their backs and the webs of their wings all mixed together, moving slowly, clogging the air. I needed more room than I used to, more space to stand in, to turn in, more light, more air.

Dean and I bought souvenirs at Disney World—a Mickey Mouse sweatshirt for me, a Mickey Mouse T-shirt for Dean. What should we get Johnny-Judy, we wondered. We bought three half-sized spoons with picture handles: Winnie the Pooh floating skyward hanging on to the string of a green balloon; Donald Duck in his sailor suit, coy, tipping his hat; Mickey with one oversized hand raised, saying, it seemed, "hi" and "stop" at the same time.

"Those aren't small enough," my Aunt Louise said. I looked at the bowl of one of the spoons, trying to imagine a mouth even too small for that. My aunt had raised three kids. She knew about sizes, about spoons, about feeding. What did I know? Not much. I had wanted the spoons to be for right away, for the first food after my own milk. "Well," I said, "they'll be good for later on."

On May 2, Dean and I made our second visit to Dr. Abram's office, this time for the amniocentesis our health center advised me to have because of my age. I had been envisioning the procedure for weeks—the needle stuck through my swollen belly. Dr. Barrie said the pain would be mild and brief, but I wasn't sure I could believe that. And what harm might we do in the process of trying to find out if our child was healthy? Fortunately for me, the placenta was not "anterior," not located at the front of my womb. Sometimes an anterior placenta made amniocentesis impossible. My fibroid didn't pose a problem either, as Dr. Barrie had feared it might. Dr. Abram assured me she could get around it. She was, Dr. Barrie said, one of the finest ultrasound diagnosticians in the state.

I tried not to think ahead to the report we would get.

We would have to wait a month or more, only to abort the pregnancy if the news turned out to be very bad.

In the small, half-lit room, Dr. Abram pressed the sensor hard against my abdomen, indenting the dome of my belly. The air in the room was cool, and the gel on my skin felt cold and sticky. Dr. Abram watched the computer-formed streaks shifting on the screen. She could keep one view of the fetus as long as she wanted by holding the sensor with a steady pressure against my belly, and she could adjust the magnification by fiddling with the knobs on the machine. She could choose, say, a close-up of the head or the empty space in the sac near the legs, or she could create a less enlarged view of the whole body resting on its curved spine in its cramped, dark cubby. The view could be held constant by Dr. Abram's steady arm and hand, but the image was alive, moving, changing. Dr. Abram would interpret the picture on the screen while Dr. Barrie inserted the needle.

I turned my face toward the wall. Dean was standing there, holding my hand. Dr. Abram's husky voice was instructing Dr. Barrie, but I didn't let myself distinguish words. I didn't want to know what was happening. I pushed everything in the room far away from me except Dean's hand. When I felt pain, a piercing sting, I began counting backwards, as Dean had told me to do. One hundred, ninety-nine, ninety-eight . . . I concentrated on the numbers, on getting each one right. I sweated into Dean's hand, gripping it like a lifeline, trying not to think about the ring of throbbing pain spreading outward from the needle as though the doctor was pushing into the center of a deep wound. The doctors were talking. Dean talking. Their voices blurred, far off. Only the numbers distinct, and the need to hold still. And then a pull up through the pain, and my thinking, I can't, I can't stay still any more. Sixty-three, sixty-two . . . "It's all over, Marion. It went real well. There's no blood in the fluid at all. It's nice and clear. How are you? Are you all right?" Dr. Barrie was talking to me. Dean was stroking my hair.

"I'm fine."

"You lie still awhile," Dr. Abram said.

"Marion, I've got to run." Dr. Barrie was talking again, leaning over me. "One of my patients is in labor at the hospital. You should rest here as long as you want. It went very well."

The second both doctors were gone, my skin felt hot everywhere and sweat soaked through my blouse. Then I was shivering and sobbing. "It hurt, Deanie, it really hurt."

"It took longer than it should have. The first syringe wasn't working. The needle was okay, but they had to switch the top part, the part that holds the fluid."

"Christ, I didn't even know."

"It's just as well you didn't. The important thing is that it's over now and you're okay."

Dr. Abram's assistant came in and handed me a photograph of the fetus—a profile of the face, with a vaguely discernible eye and a lionish nose and mouth. She handed Dean a small glass vial, test tube shaped, to carry to the Prenatal Diagnostics Lab at Mass. General. The vial was filled not with a clear liquid, as I had expected, but a yellow liquid, like urine. Dean tucked the vial into the inside pocket of his suit jacket. "This is the safest place," he assured me, giving it a pat.

We worked our way through a maze to get to the lab at Mass. General: first the unfamiliar streets surrounding the hospital, where we hunted for a place to park our car, then the stairways, elevators and corridors inside the hospital. At the lab, a receptionist took the vial from Dean and assured us that our doctor would have a result as soon as possible—four to six weeks. "We don't want to know the sex," I said.

"Be sure your doctor knows that, and remind her again when she calls you. Did you get a copy of this?" the woman asked, holding up a blue pamphlet called *Prenatal Diagnosis*.

"Yes, we did, we read it, thanks."

Indeed, I had read that booklet through several times. It talked about odds—the odds of a woman my age, and other ages, carrying a child with Down's Syndrome; the odds of amniocentesis causing a miscarriage; the odds of getting no meaningful result when the amniotic fluid is tested and needing a second test.

There was a note on the wall about the hospital's genetic counseling services. Thank God we don't need that, I said to myself. I felt sorry for the people who did.

At night sometimes after Dean fell asleep, breathing gently beside me, his back a protecting wall, a seawall I could float behind without fear, I turned to my right side and pressed my belly against his warm skin. There the baby would be, in the musky space between me and Dean, and I would press as close as I could, reaching an arm around Dean's waist to rub his stomach. And sometimes I needed enclosing myself; so I would get up, naked in the cool room, scurry around to Dean's side of the bed, and get in, trying to make myself small, fitting myself into the space in front of Dean. I would press my back against his chest and belly, push my buttocks against his nest of golden hair, his penis and balls, and pull his arm over my waist and hold his hand against the dome that held our child.

Sometimes my belly seemed to contain not just our child, but the whole of me as well. It seemed that I was curled up in that dark space, and that space was like a bubble, delicate, stretched, that might float away or burst.

My skin was thin, taut (so I imagined it); and it was permeable. I often felt like one of those shapes that has no inside or outside, and yet has both, the inside and outside edge being one. My connection to the fetus inside me connected me in turn to the world beyond my skin.

That spring, as the leaves unfolded and the flowers opened, "Now you understand," they said. "Now you know, for the first time, how we unfold, expand, recreate life."

I remember on one occasion feeling an uncanny, joyful intensity in an ordinary sight—an old yellow house in the sunlight at the top of a lawn sloping to the road. I was driving by it, and I just caught the scene for a few seconds. It was a house I had seen many times before, but now a new soul seemed to be looking at it through my eyes. The whole scene—the light on the pale yellow shingles, the drooping panicles of purple wisteria framing the door—it was mine, it came into me, as though claimed by the child inside me. The image hung in my mind as I drove, like a diamond turning in the air in a sunny room. I shared it—already shared the world—with my child.

I don't remember whose idea it was—mine or Dean's—to go out for dinner on Mother's Day. I do remember being bashful, afraid of assuming too much—superstitious.

"Do you really think I rate?" I asked Dean.

"I do. Sure you rate, look at you." He pointed to my belly. "What does Johnny-Judy think?"

I pulled in my chin, looking down, slipping my fingers back and forth over my belly, smoothing the fabric of my blouse against it. "Well, Johnny-Judy, do you think it's a good idea?"

Calling my mother to wish her a happy Mother's Day, I decided she would know: "Tell me, you're an authority. Do you think I'm entitled to a Mother's Day dinner?"

She laughed. "Oh, absolutely."

At the restaurant I kept looking around to spot the other mothers, the real ones, like my mother. Impossible as it seemed, next Mother's Day we would have an infant to tend to at dinner. "Will we bring Johnny-Judy with us next year?" My thoughts turned to babysitters and vague apprehensions about finding one, trusting one. "Is Mother's Day a day you get a sitter, or do you want your kid with you?"

"I guess it depends how sick you are of your kid. And how much of a slob you want to be." Dean waved his hand over the mess on the table, the spilled butter and busted shells from our two boiled lobsters.

I smiled.

"Hallmark will love you," Dean said. "You'll be just like all the other mothers."

Really, it was true. Already I kept picturing myself opening my first card. Pretending Johnny-Judy had picked it out. Ridiculous! What silly saying would Dean choose?

"What will my first card say?"

"How about one of those little trophies instead? You know. . . ." Dean made quotation marks with his fingers. "World's Greatest Mom."

CHAPTER 2

FETUS IN STRESS

1

It's the fourth Sunday in May and the baby and I are entering some new phase. I've been learning to expect new phases, wondering at every moment what change my body will go through next.

"How are you?" my mother asks, calling from Poughkeepsie around lunchtime.

I stand at the kitchen counter making sandwiches and feel for a second time a twinge in my abdomen and an annoying crampiness. "Great, I'm doing great. I think my hormones are shifting or something, though. I'm sort of crampy today."

"Is the baby kicking yet?"

"No, not yet, but people say some babies start a little later than others. In the next couple of weeks I should feel it."

"Maybe it has started," my friend Ann suggests, when she and her husband come for dinner with their two little boys. "It doesn't really feel like a kick. It's more like a twinge. I remember being kind of confused my first time, not knowing right away what I was feeling." She rocks Matthew in her arms, his two-month-old moon face peering around the fleshy bumper to watch his older brother's top, whirring on the floor before a broad, flat face like his own. "Once it starts, you'll wish it would stop. It can drive you crazy all night."

"I know, that's what Dean's brother's wife says, but I don't care, I just want it to start. Maybe you're right, maybe these twinges I'm feeling are kicks."

I have two photos of me that Dean took that Sunday. I almost never look at them, but I would be miserable if I lost them and I'm thankful I didn't mail one to my friend Cindy, as I had planned. I was standing barefoot on our front lawn in the afternoon sun. No rain. The grass was dry for the first time in over a week. Irises were blooming around the boulder by the driveway, brilliant gold and lavender against the gray stone, and the pieris beneath the living room window was covered with clusters of white flowers.

I posed in my newest maternity outfit, my favorite: a blue denim jumper with bronze-colored buttons holding the shoulder straps to the front yoke (this, the saleswoman had said, would be a godsend for nursing) and a red confetti-printed blouse with white collar and white cuffs. The pieris and rhododendron were a wash of white and sea-green and shadow behind me. I faced the camera and, forming a cradle of my hands, placed them under my belly, pressing against the jumper to show my roundness. This wasn't so good, Dean thought, not a natural enough pose to send to Cindy in New York to show her what I looked like pregnant. So we tried a second shot, my protruding abdomen in profile, with a three-quarter view of my face, my clasped hands resting on the shelf of my belly. That was it. That was me pregnant. I stood there on the lawn with Dean and watched my ghostlike emergence on the instant film.

"I'll keep the first one for me," I said, planning a record against the day when my body would be skinny again, forgetful of the fullness, the expectancy, the soundless, unfathomable drifting of outside in. Already I could see myself holding out the picture to a grabby, giggling, half-interested child. The child was nebulous, neither boy nor girl, but I was certain of the giggle and the preoccupation with things other than me. That was the goal, after all. The tatter of sky caught in my womb would float out again and take my child with it.

"I've been up all night," I told the nurse when I called the health center in the morning. "I couldn't go to work today." The twinge had evolved overnight into a mild, steady ache, a hum of pain against a background of cramps. "I think it must be gas. Could that hurt this much?"

"Yes, it may be gas. From what you describe, I don't see any reason to be alarmed, just call us on Thursday if you still don't feel well and we'll have you come in."

"Is it queer that there's this funny pressure when I urinate? It's hard to describe. It feels sort of swollen down there on the outside around the vagina. It actually hurts to use the muscles."

"That's not unusual, the hormones can make it feel that way. Let's wait a few days like I said and see how you're doing. If you're still in pain on Thursday, give me a call."

It was raining again. From where I lay in bed I could see the new leaves of the sugar maple and the thick gray-white light of the sky; and the crab apple, its dripping leaves pasted with white petals, its branches messy with the dried brown hearts of fallen flowers. A few pink-white blossoms still fluttered in the wet wind.

I rehearsed the phone call as though I had made a tape of it in my mind. The nurse had not shown the slightest alarm. My problem was probably gas, maybe a recurrence, in a new guise, of the discomfort of my third month, when drinking a quart of milk every day had caused gas pains so sharp that it had been difficult to walk. Perhaps even the half-quart I still drank was too much. Or perhaps my problem just came from being pregnant and couldn't be helped. There might be no cure for it beyond waiting.

Fortitude. Mine was much too great to be shaken by this pain. It had already been tested and braced by the fibroid tumor, continuing to grow, violating the baby's universe. I tried my best not to pay attention to the round mass. When I rubbed my belly, making small, soothing circles with my fingertips, I avoided the hard, uneven place. When a relative or friend pressed my abdomen, testing the heft of my new shape, I tried to keep my hands over the fibroid. When one of my aunts happened to touch it and exclaim how hard my belly was, I smiled in agreement. No one knew about the tumor except me and Dean and the doctors.

I listened to the steady rustling of rain in the trees and the thumping drip from a leaking gutter and anticipated the gradual easing of pain and my sinking into sleep. Cool, damp air blowing in through the screens touched my face and arms. I thought about the baby's room, still not a baby's room at all, but a barely used roomful of odds and ends that would have to be thrown out or stored in the basement or put in a closet. It was a small, dark room, on the back side—the west side—of the house. Dean and I had tried sleeping in it when we had first moved into the house but had finally given it up as too claustrophobic. We had settled into the front corner bedroom, slightly larger, with sunlight soaking through the curtains at dawn. The only other bedroom, the one next to ours, we had turned into an office; I liked working there, looking up from time to time at the crab apple and the spruce, and the sky over the front lawn.

Dean and I had decided that the baby's room could be a bright room too, but it needed more windows than the two it had; they were small and oddly placed, catty-corner, almost touching, one in the side wall of the house, and one in the back. In July or August we would hire someone to add a long window in the back wall, looking out at the rock garden and the tall pines. Finally the afternoon sun would be able to reach into the room through the trees. Then we would replace the dingy wallpaper left over from the former owners. We would pick out something playful. Something with four or five different colors. Bright colors. Flowers, perhaps; or ABC's; or maybe stripes.

The only alteration in the baby's room so far was the growing menagerie of stuffed creatures: the sandy-colored teddy bear Dean's mother had sent, the yellow chick with the bright orange beak from a neighbor, and the red-lipped sock monkey I had bought. I envisioned the animals on neat new shelves against the new paper. There would be a crib and a bureau and such other necessities as I couldn't yet imagine. (We had so much to do, and with only four months left.)

That night Dean worked late, and by the time he got home at ten-thirty he was exhausted. I was exhausted too, having failed to sleep at all during the day. We were both edgy, and we both needed ministering to. I suggested that we sleep separately, so Dean could avoid my restlessness in bed, and we did, after he first tried unsuccessfully to sleep beside me. He was too tired to open our foldout couch, or to move the unfolded laundry heaped on the spare bed in the baby's room, so he nestled in a sleeping bag on the living room rug.

I stand at the living room end of the hall and watch Dean sleeping, listen to his breathing, draw comfort from him. I make a silent promise not to wake him and I keep it as long as I can, holding on to it more and more desperately as the night progresses and the pain becomes hotter and more focused and no longer seems at all like gas.

I try to limp or crawl or bend or fall away from the pain. I roll from side to side on the bed, pressing my knees together like a mad cricket and gripping the sheets. I pace in monotonous circles, monotonous loops, into the bedroom, out of the bedroom, into the bedroom, out of the bedroom. I read catalogs, the same two, the same pages, over and over, over and over. I try warm baths. I slump in the tub as low as I can without letting my mouth go under, pushing the water in waves over my big belly. I stand in the hall, naked, and pray for the fire in my right side to go out.

The pale blue light begins to fill the panes of the windows and filters into the house like phosphorous, making the lampshade in the living room glow like a moth and everything in the room shimmer. When I shake Dean's arm and whisper for his help, it seems to me he sleeps afloat on a pool—a black, acid pool—where I am drowning.

I didn't know it then, but Amelia was dying.

2

"Whatever they do, don't let them make me go to the hospital."

"They can't force you to do anything you don't want. And I'll be right there with you. You're going to be all right."

Dean and I were in the car, heading to the health center.

Dr. Lamont, whom I had never met before, talked to me while I shifted position incessantly on the examining table, grimacing and whimpering. "It may be the fibroid," I heard him saying, confirming what I had begun to suspect. "I'm not sure. I don't think it's appendicitis, but we need to rule that out." He paused, looking at me, giving me a few seconds to look at him.

"I think you ought to be in the hospital. We need to get that pain under control."

I started crying. I had never been hospitalized and the prospect terrified me. I assumed I would be running the risk of some deadly mix-up. I imagined myself being wheeled into an operating room by mistake. What would they remove? One of my breasts? One of my legs? Would the baby be harmed?

Dr. Lamont was a gentle examiner, respectful of me, considerate of my pain. But he was so earnest I was suspicious. How did I know he wasn't being overzealous? How many of his patients did he catch in this trap? "Of course, you're free to go home, I can't stop you, but I think it's unwise."

At the doctor's suggestion, Dean and I went to the waiting area to think things over. "Maybe he's right," Dean said, "how can you go home like this?" I was clutching his hand, walking slowly, limping, lowering myself laboriously onto one of the lounge chairs, holding my legs outstretched. I felt as though a molten pellet was lodged in my abdomen. Sitting still had become impossible. I writhed; rocked back and forth like a retarded child; gripped the seat with my hands and raised and lowered my buttocks. Nothing worked. I was aware of the calmness of other women in other chairs, and their quietness. I couldn't stop moving, making noise, crying, whimpering, groaning. I spread my hands lightly over my swollen belly. I was scared.

While Dean was phoning his office and mine, Dr. Lamont came out to where I was sitting, and his face, looking down at me, was kind, his features large, distorted, as though I was seeing him through a fisheye lens. "How are you doing?"

"I give up. I'll go to the hospital."

On the drive to Brigham and Women's, I had this crazy feeling of wanting to roll out of myself, out of the car, away from the pain. "Try putting the seat-back down," Dean said. I lowered it as far as I could and dug my nails into the seat and watched the rain beads shimmying down the window and listened to Dean's reassurances over my moaning and crying. "I know you're scared, Marion, but I'm with you, and I'll stay right by you. You'll be all right, I know you will. You're doing the smart thing, you couldn't have gone home like this." The stores and houses and trees along the route were monotonous, blurred extensions of my pain. I was depending on Dean to interpret the world. When I walked with him to the hospital from the parking garage, leaning on his arm, moving slowly, gingerly, in spite of the heavy rain, I had no more sense of my location in Boston than I would have had if I had traveled through a tunnel from the doctor's office. I passed into the alien bustle of the hospital lobby without even noticing what the building looked like outside—its size or color or shape.

In seconds, or so it seemed, I had a plastic ID band around my wrist and I was seated in a wheelchair. A young man in a baggy green uniform was pushing me down a hall off the main lobby. I kept looking behind me to be sure Dean was following. My relief at no longer having to make any effort to move on my own disturbed and surprised me; the thought forced itself on me—I'm *that* sick.

We entered an elevator large enough for several wheelchairs and it made me feel helpless, swallowed. I wondered which floor the rooms were on that Dean and I would visit in our third trimester when we toured the delivery area. Now we'll be ahead of the game, I told myself, trying to cheer myself up. We'll know what the building is like, and Dean will know his way here; the tour will be less intimidating.

A nurse took over from the orderly and wheeled me into a room with two beds. On the bed closest to the window a white terrycloth robe lay on top of a turned-down white thermal blanket, and paper cups, magazines and greeting cards littered an oblong table alongside the bed. Tuned to an evangelist talk show, a large television, an ugly brown box on brackets, hung high on the wall facing the bed, impossible to ignore. I got out of the wheelchair with Dean's help and sat on the edge of the stripped bed nearer the door and stared at the screen, at the two men talking in Southern accents. "If they don't get me a private room, I'm leaving. How the hell am I supposed to sleep in here? I'd be better off at home."

A toilet flushed, and a young woman, twenty-five or so, big-bellied like me, emerged from behind the wooden door near the window. I answered her "hello" in a blank, unfriendly voice. I didn't want her asking me any questions. Sitting in a chair by her bed, she worked the television's remote control, and with a clicking sound the screen shifted to some kind of quiz show. Jingly music. Applause.

By the time the nurse came in, I was fighting back tears, muttering to Dean about leaving the hospital. But the problem dissolved. "Your doctor requested a private room, is that right? We can move you now, Marion. Just have a seat in the wheelchair again and we'll get you settled. We don't have to go far, just two doors down."

In minutes I was in bed wearing a blue and white striped hospital johnny in a room of my own. I had finally come to rest, nudged to safety like a child. I had no more sense of my location within the hospital than I had of the hospital's location in Boston. I had glimpsed corridors leading to more corridors, doorways followed by more doorways, but they were unanchored scraps of space. I hadn't even noticed what floor the elevator had stopped at. I had no orientation and I needed none. I lay down gratefully between the sheets and waited for help. The nurse brought me the Percodan Dr. Lamont had ordered, and I took it, though I still feared, in spite of his assurances to the contrary, that the drug would harm the baby.

Dean moved around the room trying to make it comfortable for me, trying to anticipate my wishes. He opened the curtains, and it cheered me to see a window as long as my bed. Except for the heating-air conditioning unit forming a sort of windowsill, the window filled the wall to my right. The view was ugly: the top floors of the parking garage, and a wet stretch of hospital roof interrupted only by a looming tower, windowless, like a factory smokestack without smoke, some kind of exhaust system, I assumed, necessary for some complicated hospital purpose. I was glad I could see something of the world outside, even something grim. The tower was a focus beyond my pain, benignly indifferent, and so were the stick figures going to and from their cars on the parking lot roof.

Dean opened and closed the blinds, thin white slats encased in the double-paned window. "Look how these work." He turned a knob on the inside pane of glass. "How's that? Too light for you?" Dean tilted the slats again, reducing the light in the room but leaving me my view of the dreary day.

"I like that, it's perfect, thanks."

The only decoration in the room was the fabric of the curtains, off-white with an abstract design in bright red, green, blue and yellow. I liked the repeating pattern, squiggly vertical lines I could trace up and down, interrupted by broken rings, Life Savers sucked by invisible mouths into colorful "c's." The bed had no bedspread, only a white thermal blanket; and the walls, vanilla-colored, were plain, without any pictures. A cork bulletin board in a steel frame hung on the wall opposite me. Dean read and removed the two printed notices tacked to it and stored them underneath my sandals at the bottom of the metal clothes locker. A few feet from the bulletin board, closer to the window and at a right angle to it, was a heavy-looking door of blond wood. Dean opened it. "You've got your own bathroom. Let's see how it works. I'll take a leak." I liked hearing him peeing in there, an intimate, homey sound, a sound that made it Dean's room as well as mine. "You've got a shower," he said when he came out, "and another sink."

There was a sink in the room, too, in an L-shaped nook cut in the wall opposite me to the left of the bulletin board. The sink was set diagonally into the angle of the nook and it had a formica counter around it. Dean pulled a toothbrush out of a blue plastic pail on the counter and held it up, then a plastic bottle of Keri Lotion. "What's that for?" I mumbled into the pillow, which had a plastic cover inside the pillow case and crinkled under my head.

"I don't know." Dean shrugged, squeezing some of the white lotion into his hands and rubbing it into mine.

"It feels nice." I spoke with effort, distracted by the burning pain and by the drowsiness I was beginning to feel. Dean arranged the toothbrush and lotion and a bar of Dial soap on the sink counter and put the pail inside the locker. "Keep the pail out. I like it."

I focused my eyes on the pail for a few seconds and then closed them, feeling as though sleep might be within reach, finally, after more than forty-eight hours. "Go on to work now," I said, almost inaudibly, thinking how fortunate it was that I didn't have a job like Dean's. With my job it would hardly matter if I was out for a few days.

"Are you sure it's okay? I won't go if you don't want me to." Dean leaned over the bed and kissed me. "Would you like me to lower the bed?"

"Yes, please, that's a good idea."

Dean figured out how to lower the angle of the upper part of the bed, and after adjusting me downward several inches he moved the cord so that the control panel with the red button would be easily within my reach. "Just press this if you want to sit up more. And here, let's clip the nurses' button right here, under your pillow. Don't you be reluctant to use it. I know you."

I tried the button for the bed, raising and lowering my back and head. "I wish they gave you more blankets."

Dean raised his hand in a gesture that said "no problem" and left the room, returning with two more of the white thermal blankets. "There's a whole stack of them right outside."

"Do they have any decent pillows? Listen to this thing." I moved my head, and the pillow made a crackling sound, like crumpled cellophane.

"They've all got plastic covers," Dean reported from the doorway. "I'll get your mushy one from the car."

"Don't bother about it now. Bring it after work." Dean agreed and we hugged and kissed good-bye, but in fifteen minutes he was back with the pillow I had brought for the car ride to the health center. He held out the limp down pillow in the faded yellow case and laughed. "You call this a pillow? Look at this thing, it looks like it died."

I smiled. "Thanks."

"This will help, too." Dean showed me a makeshift pillow, two thermal blankets in a hospital pillow case. "Pretty clever, huh, Frog?"

"Thanks." I kissed Dean's hand. "You go on to work now."

"I'll be back around six. And I know what this room needs, I know what I'm gonna get for it."

I wondered about that as I fell off to sleep, thinking, too, about pails and shovels and beaches and what a great dad Dean was going to make.

I hear a door close—a pneumatic hiss, a settling of wood. They don't want me to hear it. They don't want me to call them back. It's raining in the room, water rising around the bed in the dark, lapping against it.

Something smells good, something floating near me on the surface of the water.

I open my eyes. White sheets, white blankets. I'm in the hospital. The pain. The baby. Someone's put a tray of food on the table by the bed. It's lunchtime. I've only slept an hour or so.

I wanted to sit up. I was hungry. The bed whirred beneath me when I pressed the button, but the raised mattress only sloped annoyingly behind my head. I would need to boost myself up. The pain, though, was a warning, a threat, a menacing concentration of energy, like the eye of a bull in a field. I pushed against the mattress with my elbows, leaned my weight on them, walked them behind me, first one, then both. The eye was watching. I shifted to my hands, propping myself higher, pushing against the mattress, dragging myself up until I was sitting. But the three pillows flopped into the space behind me, bunching up so I couldn't lean back. I lowered the bed, rearranged the pillows, dragged myself higher on the mattress so there wouldn't be any gap behind me this time, then raised the bed again, reaching back to hold the pillows in place. *So that's how it's done.* My body felt heavy, thick, weak. The glowering eye never looked away. I swung the hinged table over the bed, pulling it in front of me above my cumbersome belly, and lifted the plastic lid off the lunch plate with curiosity. I was glad for the diverting details of mealtime—the good tastes and smells, the novelty of being waited on in bed.

A woman wearing a white doctor's coat over a lavender dress came in to see me while I was eating. Her face had a scrubbed, motherly look. She belonged on a sunny lawn, with kids pressing against her legs, tugging at the hem of her dress. From the way she stood at the foot of the bed, I could tell she wouldn't be staying long. "Hi, I'm Dr. O'Shea." She offered me her words as though they were solid objects I could hold on to. "Dr. Barrie couldn't be here to admit you, but she'll be in to see you sometime this afternoon, probably late afternoon. Did you sleep?"

My voice when I answered was thick and slow, the way my body felt, and I had to think hard about what I wanted to say. "I think I need help getting to the bathroom."

"The nurse will help you. I'll tell her."

A few minutes after the doctor left, I reached under my pillow for the cord clipped to the sheet and pressed the red button at the end of the thumb-sized plastic piece. The speaker in the wall above the bed clicked and I waited for the nurse's voice, expecting her to tell me she was busy, but a nurse appeared in the half-open doorway. "I was just about to come in," she said, in a thin, friendly voice, helpful but not pushy. Her skin was freckled, and her shoulder-length hair was the color of damp sand. She entered the room with silent, bouncy steps, and the thick gum soles of her nurse's shoes made her seem sturdy, even though she was skinny and quite young. She stood by my bed, close enough to touch.

"Thanks, I need to use the bathroom but I feel so sick. Could you just stay in the room while I go?" I sounded as though my mouth was filled with wool. I started apologizing for being a bother, but the nurse shushed me, leaning over to help me out of bed.

"You shouldn't get up by yourself. Just call me or one of the others. That's what we're here for." I leaned hard on her arm as she walked with me to the door of the bathroom. "My name's Tina."

When I came out of the bathroom, Tina was changing my sheets, which were soaked with sweat. She helped lower me into the big chair by the bedside—a green vinyl monstrosity which I liked nonetheless because of its homey wing chair shape and size. I waited, slouched down with my legs straight out in front of me and my right arm gripping the arm of the chair to lift some of the weight off my abdomen and onto my left side. Tucking the clean new sheets under the mattress, Tina moved quickly, deftly. "I'll just be a minute more, Marion." She made the bed with an extra sheet over the bottom one, a wide band across the middle of the bed, so there would be two sheets to soak up my sweat instead of one. "There, now, let me help you in." I perched at the edge of the chair, my belly rounded like a turtle's back, and pushed slowly with my right hand while Tina slipped a supporting arm around my waist and steadied me as I stood up. I closed my eyes for a second, feeling dizzy and sick to my stomach, and put my left arm around Tina's waist. She patted my left hand with hers and inched with me toward the bed as though nothing in the world mattered except getting me safely across those few feet of space.

Once I was in bed and Tina had helped me arrange my pillows the way I wanted them, she took my temperature and blood pressure and checked the fetal heartbeat. With the covers turned down and my hospital johnny pulled up to my chest, my bare belly seemed to fill the room. Tina listened and smiled. "It's nice and strong."

"Shall I close the door?" she asked when she was through.

In the corridor, an intercom called like a conscience, "Dr. Hanson, Dr. Hanson." A nurse near my door but not visible to me laughed at something. Through the doorway, I could see a piece of the corridor, just a few feet of cream-colored space, and I could see part of the open doorway to another room. "I'd like the door open, please, just halfway." Tina pulled the door after her until the opening was just the width of her back, and it automatically held. More than the tray of food or the intercom button, the open doorway helped keep me from feeling cut off, forgotten.

I lay there on my left side, wondering what terrible thing would happen to me and to the baby if the pain didn't go away. "Johnny-Judy," I mumbled, closing my eyes. The Demerol shot the nurse had given me made the pain just bearable enough so sleep seemed possible and I began to drowse again.

When I heard Dr. Barrie talking to me, I gave up my sleep reluctantly and opened my eyes. Outside, the sky was dark gray; a dismal mist hung about the tower. "What time is it?"

"About four o'clock." Dr. Barrie had bluish half-moons of fatigue under her eyes. "I'm sorry this is happening to you."

"I'm scared."

"I know, we've got to get this pain under control."

"Why is this happening?"

"I wish I could tell you, but I don't know."

"Is it my appendix?"

"No. We've ruled that out. I'd say it's the fibroid."

Dr. Barrie had me bare my belly and she pressed gently on it, here and there, her gray eyes concentrating, connected to her fingertips it seemed. She pushed into the hard area where the tumor was. I howled like a dog.

"I'm sorry, I won't press there anymore."

"It is the fibroid, isn't it?"

"Yes, I'd say it's becoming necrotic."

"What's that mean?"

"It's not getting the blood supply it wants. I don't know why."

"Will I need an operation?"

"I don't want to operate while you're pregnant. I just want to get you through this until you deliver. That's why it's so important for us to get the pain under control. We need to make it bearable for you. When you're farther along, perhaps we can induce labor, but not now, it's much too early. After you deliver, the tumor should shrink, but if it doesn't, then yes, I would have to operate. I'm going to send you for an ultrasound tomorrow to have a look at the baby. I'll stop in to see you again tonight." Dr. Barrie's studied enunciation of each word betrayed her worry. I'm sure she wanted it to. She was preparing me, though for what even she didn't know.

I was sitting up eating dinner when Dean walked in and stood his briefcase on the floor. It fell over with a rattle. He looked at it and groaned. "I'm beat."

I held up my arms in a mock hug and he came to the bed and leaned over me, smelling good, his hair tickling my face. "I love you," we both said.

"What's in the bag?" Dean had laid a big paper bag at the foot of the bed.

"Close your eyes. Keep them closed. Keep them closed."

I put down my fork and closed my eyes, listening to the sound of paper being handled and smoothed, and tape—Scotch tape, it sounded like—being cut. "Okay, open."

A poster was taped to the bathroom door—a neat rectangle of bright color against the pale wood. Charlie Brown was hanging upside down in a tree, entwined in the string of a kite stuck in the branches. "Why me?" the poster said under Charlie Brown's inverted round head.

I was glad to have the poster. It gave the room a homey touch, and that evening, after Dean had gone home, it was a reminder of him—his attentiveness, his penchant for odd little surprises. But I felt bad for Charlie Brown. The pickle he was in worried me, the way slapstick comedy always does. And his question, "Why me?"—I didn't like seeing it there, written out. For him it was funny, but not for me. When I asked it, I felt angry; I imagined hundreds, thousands, of women whose pregnancies were trouble-free. "Why me? Why not one of them?"

The next morning, Wednesday, a man wearing white

pants and a loose white shirt appeared in the doorway of my room. "Your wheelchair's ready," he said.

"What?" I felt frightened.

"You're having an ultrasound. Didn't your doctor tell you?" The man's voice was gentle and he took charge calmly.

Tina came in to help me out of bed, instructing me to sit on the edge to ease the dizziness before I stood up. She and the man helped me into the wheelchair, and he moved the footrests into place. Then the walls and doorways along the corridor began moving past me and I felt as though I might vomit. The wheels rolled over a bump in the hard floor and my right side throbbed like the beaten center of a gong. "Slower, please, slower," I moaned, holding up a hand. The man slowed down, and he eased me carefully over the threshold of the elevator.

"You let me know now if I'm hurting you." I concentrated on his voice and on his strong brown arms reaching to release the brake as he wheeled me out of the elevator into the basement corridor. His pressure on the back of the chair was firm, holding me back now as much as pushing me forward, slowing the chair almost to a halt around corners and over bumps. He anticipated these dangers the way a commuting driver anticipates curves and potholes in the road. "Easy does it. There, now, is that slow enough? Don't forget, you tell me now if I'm hurting you."

The wide corridor moved past me with the placeless inevitability of a labyrinth in a dream, and everything I saw was oddly remote, as though I looked out from a tank filled with water. I felt myself blurring and receding from the world, and increasingly I feared that I might go unnoticed and forgotten. Anyone who spoke to me or touched me was important, looming at me as though through parted waters, and if the voice or touch was kind I wanted to cling to it. "Thanks," I told the man. "I'm sorry to be such a problem."

"Allll-most there."

We passed a sign on the corridor wall: RADIOLOGY, and the man stopped alongside a wide opening into a brightly lighted room.

"I can't have X rays," I said, struggling to sound coherent. "I'm pregnant."

"They know that, you're here for ultrasound. It's in the same department. You're okay." He was slow and gentle turning my wheelchair to face the room and I was suddenly afraid of his leaving me as he positioned my wheelchair so that it was one of four arranged in a row across the middle of the room. In each chair a patient sat. The room smelled like sweat and stale breath and plastic and rubber. The wheelchairs faced a high wooden desk set apart like a speaker's podium across about five feet of empty space. We might have been prisoners waiting for a forced lecture; weak, wary. "There'll be a little wait," the man said to me after talking to the administrator at the desk. "I'll be back for you."

"How long will I have to wait? It hurts so much."

"Not too long I shouldn't think. The room we're waiting for is occupied now, but you're the next one in." The man left, trying to reassure me with a backward glance from the doorway.

There was a sign on the desk: IF YOU ARE PREGNANT TELL THE ATTENDANT. I called across the room to the man behind the desk. "Excuse me, sir, I want to be sure you know I'm pregnant. I can't have any X rays."

The man examined a tray of standing files. "Wasserman? Don't worry, Miss, it's all down here." He wasn't rude, but he wasn't friendly either.

I looked at the woman next to me on my right. She was old, with brown blotches on her frail face. She tilted her head to look at me and each of her eyes seemed drawn to a stabbing point; then she shut them and her head fell forward. Every few seconds she winced. An orderly came in and moved me back and over, so now I was in the second row, behind the old woman, and a stretcher was moved in where I had been, the patient's gray face lined up between the old woman and another patient in the first row. The lower half of the stretcher was next to me on my left, and I stared for a moment at the sheet-covered legs hemming me in. More stretchers were lined up along the wall behind me. I wondered what diseases these people had and I felt a panicky fear of contamination. I rubbed my belly softly, in tiny circles. Cut off now from the desk, I didn't have the courage to call out over the patients in the front row to ask how much longer I would have to wait.

The orderly returned, pushing a wheelchair with a man in it whose right leg stuck out in front of him, oddly bent and bony up to the knee and hidden from knee to groin in a heavy-looking cast. The room had become so crowded with stretchers and chairs that the orderly, a short man with close-cropped dark hair and a square mouth, stood near the doorway, looking in, as though searching for an empty seat in a crowded theater. There was no space for the man with the bad leg, so the orderly began reorganizing the patients, moving the stretcher with the gray-colored man, who was breathing heavily, gasping almost, his eyes weak but watchful. Soon the man's left arm was inches from my face, a clear liquid dripping slowly into it from a plastic bag on a pole. The orderly got behind my chair to move me again, fiddling awkwardly with the brake, jerking the chair. The throbbing in my abdomen intensified, nauseating, dizzying. The orderly said nothing to me—the chair might as well have been empty.

"Leave her," a voice snapped. The man who had brought me from my room had returned. I stifled the urge to weep—a familiar face, an ally. "Dr. Burke is ready for you. I'm sorry it took so long."

As I lay on the examining table in a large, mostly

empty, partially darkened room, my hospital johnny pulled up above my belly, I was glad the man I liked had stayed in the room. Lewis, the doctor called him. When I complained of being cold, he spread a blanket over my legs.

Dr. Burke pressed on my belly with the sensor, careful to avoid the fibroid, which I covered protectively with a cupped hand. She had short brown hair that hung straight down like a curtain about her face when she leaned forward, and she smelled faintly and pleasantly of lilac perfume. I was sure she was married and had several children. She watched the screen, which I could see too, displaying my child. I asked if the heart was beating okay and she said yes. She never betrayed, in her eyes or her voice, that anything was wrong.

After five or ten minutes of pictures, and a few minutes for me to pee, Lewis wheeled me—so slowly that it must have looked as though he too was controlled, his movements restricted, by pain—back through the labyrinth of basement corridors, into, then out of, the vaultlike elevator, through more corridors, past more rooms, past room numbers and room names, past wheelchairs lined up empty somewhere in the hall, back to my room, my cocoon of sheets and blankets and pillows. Tina helped me in and I fell asleep crying. The gray man's rheumy eyes and the baby's tiny legs were scrambling kaleidoscopically on a giant screen.

3

It was after four o'clock. There was no wall clock in the room, but I could tell the time easily now because Dean had come to visit me early in the morning on his way to work and had brought a traveling clock for my table. He had also brought me a radio, which I wasn't supposed to have according to hospital rules but which the nurses were willing to overlook. I turned the radio on now and a saxophone tooted intricately beyond my fuzziness. When Dr. Barrie appeared in the doorway, I lowered the sound, and the tooting continued, faintly, like a symptom she might turn to. She stood alongside the bed, sympathy making her pale, madonna face lean towards me, alert and protective as in a dream.

"The good news is your amniocentesis report came today and it shows nothing abnormal." On "good" her voice was suspiciously eager, and she paused too long between phrases and at the end of the sentence. She was offering me comfort; something was wrong; this "good news, bad news" was not a joke.

"The bad news is the ultrasound you had today was alarming. The fetus is in stress."

I struggled to concentrate on her round-toned voice. There's a sad, gentle quality to it (always, even when she's laughing); it reminds me of the clarinet my brother used to play. "Fetus in stress." The words told me nothing, except: this is not good. Then I heard an odd-sounding word: "hydrops." It made me think confusedly of Hydrox and eyedrops. And for some reason it made me think of white mushrooms, tiny ones in the woods. "The baby is anemic . . . very serious . . . the ultrasound shows abnormal fluid retention under the skin of the head and abdomen." And then I heard an "e" sound caught at the beginning of a medical term, a common term I knew I should know the meaning of— "eczema," or "edema."

"What does stress mean? What do you mean, the fetus is in stress?" My voice was quavering.

Doctor Barrie explained: my child would be born a vegetable. She or he would be in pain, mentally defective, blind and deaf, unable to survive much more than a year—if born alive.

"Why is this happening?"

"I don't know, but I'll be consulting with Dr. Mertz, the fetal medicine specialist here at the hospital. He may have a theory."

"Could it be the drugs I've been taking?"

"No, it's definitely not the drugs. You can feel certain of that."

"Could it be toxoplasmosis? I tried to be careful, but you know, I do so much gardening, even with gloves on. . . ."

Dr. Barrie cut me off. "Marion, you've been a perfect mother-to-be, cautious about all the right things. No one could have done more. Whatever the cause is, it's not anything you did or didn't do."

"I feel overwhelmed." I was sobbing.

"So do I."

When Dr. Barrie was gone, I lay staring at the hospital tower, at its unbroken smoothness and roundness. Had I misunderstood? Was it possible, was it really possible? I needed to speak to Dean, but I struggled against calling him at work. Give him the afternoon, I told myself, give him these few hours of not knowing.

When he arrived, he kissed me before sinking into the armchair beside my bed. He took his glasses off and rubbed his eyes. Without his glasses on, he looked like a sleepy boy. "How do you like your poster?" he asked.

"Oh, I do, it cheers up the room. It makes me think of you."

"What's the matter? Has it been a bad day?"

"Very bad, I'm afraid. I have to tell you, we got some bad news today, Dean." And then I told him quickly, the little that I knew.

He leaned forward, his elbows on his knees, his face in his hands. Tall as he is, he looked cut down, beaten, leaning forward like that.

"You must mean edema," he said after a while, "not eczema."

"That's when you get all blown up, right?"

"With fluid, yes."

"I guess you're right, that's what she said. I'm scared, Deanie."

"I know, but you're gonna be all right, even if our baby isn't."

"Promise?"

"Promise."

Then I started sobbing again. "It's like a nightmare. It's the worst possible news we could get."

"No it isn't." Dean was sitting on the bed now, holding my hands in his. "It's terrible, terrible news, but it's not the worst, because you're going to be okay and that's the most important thing. You mustn't forget that."

Dr. Barrie entered the room, followed by a woman in a blue uniform who slapped a dinner tray onto my table without looking at me or Dean. "Thank you," I said to her retreating back.

"Not too pleasant," Dr. Barrie observed.

"I'm getting used to it. The food staff and the cleaning staff, they act like I'm not even here. It's the nurses and doctors who are nice."

"Hey, better that way than the other way around," Dean said.

Dr. Barrie laughed. She moved a straight-backed chair from its usual place by the sink and sat down close to me and Dean. Her eyes, loving and pitying, told me I was right—there was no hope.

"I spoke to Dr. Mertz. He's not encouraging, but we would like the fetal cardiologist to look at you tomorrow."

"Does it matter what they find?" Dean asked. "Can they do anything to turn things around?"

"That would be unlikely, even if they do discover a heart problem. There's little or nothing that can be done, though we would like to know why this condition exists."

"Are you sure it had nothing to do with Marion's pain killers?"

"Absolutely sure."

"It's not fair." Dean reached for my hand.

"No," said Dr. Barrie, "it isn't." She sat with us in silence for a few minutes. In her summer blouse and plain, khaki-colored skirt, she looked like a visiting friend or relative rather than a doctor.

"Don't let your dinner get cold," she said finally, getting up. "Dean, you might be here early tomorrow to help Marion travel to her test. I don't want her having a bad time, like she did today getting to radiology. I think it would help to have you with her."

The doctor gone, Dean and I looked at each other, saying nothing. I ignored the tray of food.

Like wanderers in a cave, we groped for some place to rest, some ledge where we could sit down in the darkness instead of moving through it. We both came to the same place, and one of us—I don't remember who—spoke first. "Do you think what they're telling us is so bad . . . do you think we should be considering an abortion?"

"Yes. Yes I do."

Dean came to see me around breakfast time the next morning, following the new routine he had established for himself, but this day he stayed instead of going on to work. While he sat in the armchair reading the morning paper, Esther, one of the nurses, came in for the periodic check of my temperature and blood pressure and the baby's heartbeat. I bared my abdomen and she rubbed on the jelly and pressed the sensor against my skin. I cupped a hand over the fibroid. "Don't press here."

"I'll try." Pushing the monitor hard against my skin, she tightened her thin lips together as though to keep them from pulling back into a snarl. "I can't find it," she complained, pressing farther to the right. "Baby may be positioned in such a way that I'll have to try over the fibroid." (I couldn't stand the way she said "Baby.")

"No, it will hurt too much, and anyway that's not where the heartbeat has been."

"The location can change."

She wore a big, plain cross around her neck, like a nun. Twice, the day before, she had invited me to pray with her, and twice I had turned her down. The second rejection embarrassed us both. Her back stiffened as she replied, "Well, of course, if you don't want to . . ." After that she had stopped trying to comfort me, stopped appealing to my faith. ("God never gave anyone a cross he couldn't bear," she had told me earlier. I had found myself wondering how she applied that notion to suicides.)

Now she moved the sensor lower and pressed hard again, looking tense, like a child on the toilet; my abdomen was her adversary.

"This is silly," Dean said, standing up from the armchair, looking down on Esther's bent form. "You ought to give up." She scowled at him, but timidly, as though wondering if he might bodily prevent her from continuing.

"The wheelchair is here," announced the nurse supervisor, appearing in the doorway like a deus ex machina.

"I can't get a heartbeat."

"Well, forget it." The nurse put a peeved emphasis on "forget." "They'll find it in cardiology, don't worry about it now."

"Well, I might have found it if you'd have let me." Esther fairly spit the words at me. She walked out to wheel in the chair, and while her back was turned Dean gave her the finger.

It was strange being wheeled to a destination I couldn't put a name to. Something to do with "children." Children's Hospital? Children's Inn? Dean was confused about the name too, but he told me it didn't matter because the orderly would get us to the right place. I was being wheeled through a maze of corridors, in and out of freight-sized elevators, down steep rubber-treaded ramps, through swinging doors that made me think of restaurant kitchens but that only led to more corridors, more ramps. I kept looking back to be sure Dean wasn't falling too far behind. As long as he was with me, being lost or forgotten was impossible; he gave me an identity in the world of the not-sick.

When the orderly stopped, we were in a narrow vestibule where several children and their parents sat in chairs along the walls. The scene looked reassuringly like any doctor's waiting room. Next to the water cooler a little boy knelt at a yellow plastic table, building a tower out of wooden blocks. None of the children looked dramatically ill as I had imagined they would.

A pregnant woman, farther along than I, probably in her seventh or eighth month, wearing a white doctor's coat over a blue maternity dress, came out of a room off the waiting area and spoke to the nurse at the reception desk in a low voice. I envied her her maternity dress. This would be my third day wearing a hospital johnny and my purple bathrobe. (Not that my maternity dresses would seem right any more. Where was the "maternity" now? What was the point of these damned tests anyway?)

The doctor disappeared behind the same door she had come out of, and when the nurse stepped towards me I was hopeful that the tests would be done immediately. The burning in my abdomen made waiting nearly unbearable. I shifted constantly in the wheelchair, whimpering. I longed to be back in my room, lying in my bed. "Marion, I'm afraid you'll have to wait awhile. Dr. Petter and Dr. Rajabi are still with another patient."

"She's in bad pain," Dean protested, and I wished his anger could make them hurry. "Why did they get us down here so early?"

The nurse ignored the question. "You can wait in here." She pushed my wheelchair into a small examining room.

"I have to use the bathroom." The pain was spreading, so that even my bladder seemed to burn. The last shot of Demerol was wearing off—not enough to unslur my speech or clear my mind—but enough for the pain to intensify. In the bathroom the nurse had to help me out of the wheelchair. She came in again when I called her and supported me as I maneuvered back into the chair, unable to bear any weight on my right leg. Reaching the metal plate on the wall to flush the toilet was impossible. The nurse did it for me, and I marveled at her matter-of-fact, undisgusted acceptance of my helplessness.

Dean was waiting for me in the examining room, sitting up on the paper-covered table that ran the short length of the room along one wall like a window seat without a window; he was sitting awkwardly, as though embarrassed to get too comfortable, leaning his head against one of the end walls but keeping his body at an angle, looking like an oversized doll tipped over on a shelf. "Why don't you lie down? You look exhausted. I don't want the table, I'm better off staying in the wheelchair."

"No, I couldn't. I'd fall asleep, and anyhow I'd feel funny."

"You shouldn't feel funny, nobody here will mind." But Dean stayed as he was, leaning his head against the wall.

"I can't wait much longer," I whimpered, my eyes filling with tears, "it hurts too much."

After a few more minutes Dean went to speak to the nurse, and while I waited I searched for distraction in the clutter of children's things—a Big Bird doll; a mobile with fuzzy blue bunnies stirring slightly in the stale air; a child's crayon drawing of a green spider, and another of a face sticking out a long red tongue. I stuck my tongue out at the crooked, angry face and let myself cry.

"They're ready for us," said Dean, coming back into the room. He picked up the briefcase he had brought along in the hope of getting some work done. "This sure was silly to bring. How are you doing?" He touched my cheek where it was wet. "Are you all right?"

"I'm just feeling sorry for myself. Let's get this over with."

The room where the doctors were waiting was crowded with equipment, more equipment than I had come to expect for an ultrasound examination. It had the claustrophobic, cavelike look of a media buff's hide-out, crammed with boxy consoles, screens, and heavy cables, leaving little room for people. Squeezing the wheelchair into the room was impossible, so Dean helped me out of the chair at the door. He and Dr. Rajabi had to lift me onto the thinly padded surface of the examining table, which was high up, running the width of the room against the innermost wall. Because of the fibroid, I wanted to lie on my left side with my knees bent, but Dr. Rajabi asked if I could try to lie on my back. This I managed with a pillow under my knees, but I gripped Dean's hand for comfort from the pain.

"Just don't press me here," I told Dr. Rajabi, indicating the location of the fibroid. "It's excruciating if you press it."

An Indian man with a thin face and dark, anxious eyes, Dr. Rajabi looked at me as though I had a bomb under me that might go off shattering us all. "We'll try managing without it," he said, lifting the johnny and lowering my underwear off my belly and smearing my abdomen with gel.

Dr. Petter, the pregnant doctor I had seen in the vestibule, shut off the overhead lights and turned on the ultrasound monitor, and Dr. Rajabi began pressing the cold metal of the sensor against my skin.

"There it is!" Dr. Petter said, with a squeak of delight in her voice. "Has Daddy seen the baby?"

I could scarcely believe I had heard her correctly. For Christ's sake, I thought, she knows why we're here.

She knows. I started sobbing. "I don't want to look anymore. I don't want to see the baby."

Dean said nothing to Dr. Petter, but he put his face close to mine. "Hey, that's okay, we don't have to look anymore. I'm not looking either."

The two doctors hung back silently, waiting for me to calm down, and then Dr. Rajabi came forward and began pressing my belly again. For the next ten minutes or so, the doctors exchanged frustrated comments while Dr. Rajabi kept shifting the pressure on my abdomen, holding the sensor everywhere but directly on the fibroid. "We're not getting what we want," he said finally.

"I'm sorry I can't help more, I'm really sorry."

"Can I try over the fibroid, Marion, not too hard?" I hesitated, then agreed, hoping to get the test over with. I knew Dr. Rajabi wanted a clear image of the baby's heart and this might be the only way to get it. I clenched one of Dean's arms with both my hands. Dr. Rajabi moved the sensor over the center of the tumor and pressed.

. . . I was shrieking, Dean was shouting, "Leave her alone! Forget your test! We don't want the goddamned test, do you understand?" (When I recall it, there's a spike driven through the tumor and I'm lifting through the ceiling of the room.)

The doctors said nothing.

Seated again in the wheelchair, I felt like a failure.

"Forget the stupid test," Dean told me. "What good would it do anyway? We all know it's academic. It's for the doctors. Who's thinking of you?"

In the afternoon, after Dean had gone to work, Dr. Lamont stopped in to see me. For several hours I had been alone, unable to sleep, unable to fight off the sense that the coming days were impenetrably shrouded, the sense that time and all expectancy were forever clotted and clogged.

I was pleased to see Dr. Lamont—his sympathetic, bovine eyes, his wiry competence; and I told him about the cardiology test.

"It sounds like they lost sight of who the patient is."

Then I told him about Esther.

"I hate to put in a complaint about her," he said, "because you'll still be seeing her when she comes around and it will just be awkward for you."

I nodded.

"How about if no one takes the heartbeat anymore but me or Dr. Barrie? No nurses. I'll write a note on your chart."

"That never occurred to me. Thank you."

In the evening, Dr. Mertz, the fetal medicine specialist, came with Dr. Barrie to talk to me and Dean. Dr. Mertz admitted to being bewildered by what was happening. No hypothesis fit the facts, and the cardiology exam had produced no clues. "All I can tell you," he said, "is that this is a random occurrence. There's no reason it should happen to you again in another pregnancy. None." He described what the baby would be like, using the words Dr. Barrie had used. Vegetable. Blind. Deaf. There was no way of changing this, he said, no remedy. Nothing they could do to make the baby well. When he finished speaking, a long silence filled my room. His penetrating eyes looked at me as though we were both refugees from some happier time and place.

Finally, one of us, Dean or I, broke the silence: "Would it be sensible for us to consider an abortion?"

"Yes it would," said Dr. Barrie, and Dr. Mertz nodded.

Dr. Barrie explained what a "termination" of my pregnancy would involve. I would be given something to induce contractions; if the drug worked well, the fetus would be expelled as in a natural delivery. Because of its immaturity, the fetus would be incapable of living outside the womb, its lungs not yet able to function. If the drug didn't work well, the fetus would have to be "extracted." This would mean cutting up the fetus inside my womb and then extracting the pieces.

Our baby was doomed, either to this premature assault or to birth into an agonizing vegetable existence that wouldn't last more than a year. That was the choice. And the longer the pregnancy continued, the larger the fibroid would grow. Dr. Barrie had told me it was already the size of a large grapefruit, and if the pain were to become so great as to require operating during pregnancy there would be a serious risk of my hemorrhaging.

I looked at Dean. He was slumped in the chair, his long arms resting heavily on his thighs, his face raised just enough for his eyes to look wearily back at me. He nodded. We were of one mind.

"We want you to do it," I said. "When will it be?"

"I'll reserve the delivery room for Sunday. We'll give you the prostaglandins on Saturday."

Three days. In three days the baby would be gone.

After Dean went home that night, I called my parents. They knew I was in the hospital, but they didn't know yet about the fetus not being normal. The phone rang a long time, and it was my father who finally answered. "Mother's out with the dog," he said. "No, wait a minute, she's just coming in."

"Ask her to pick up the extension."

A few seconds passed and then I heard my mother's voice, filled with anxiety for me. "I'm on. How are you?"

"Can you understand me? I know I sound out of it."

"We can understand you."

"We're going to abort the baby. There's something terrible wrong with it. They don't know why."

There was a silence. Then, "Do you want me to come out there?" my mother asked. "I'll come right out. If Dad can't make the trip, I'll come alone." My father, seventy-five years old and in ill health, had difficulty traveling; even with my mother driving, the five-hour car ride from Poughkeepsie to Boston was an ordeal for him.

"Thanks, I know you want to help. I appreciate that. But it's hard for you to get here. Let's wait awhile." I wished, for my mother's sake, that I could have wanted my parents beside me then. But I didn't. I knew I would feel more frightened, not less, if they were there. Their distress would add to mine. "I'd really rather just be alone with Dean. That's what we need right now."

On Friday Dean again spent the morning at the hospital. This time he stayed to accompany me to the radiology department where we were both to view the fetus through ultrasound. The doctors wanted us to see the physical evidence that our child was diseased. Neither one of us wanted to look anymore at the clear fetal image, the tiny heart pumping and pumping, but we agreed.

A nurse I hadn't seen before came into my room a half hour before the scheduled test to instruct me to drink at least three glasses of water or juice to fill my bladder for the sonogram.

"I don't need a full bladder," I told her. "I'm in my fifth month. I've had ultrasound without it several times, just yesterday in fact."

The nurse insisted, and I felt too weak to argue. "All right, maybe one glass."

"No! Nothing!" Dean glowered at the nurse. "That's it. She's not going to be tortured."

"Okay, okay, forget about it."

In the hospital basement, the radiology receptionist, presiding over a large empty waiting room different from the one I had been in on Wednesday, told me to drink some water from the cooler. "As many cups as you can." I let Dean refuse for me; then he helped me out of the wheelchair and into the bathroom. It was getting so that every half hour or so I had to pee.

The doctor who explained the sonogram to us was one I hadn't met before. Dean and I warned him immediately that if he could tell our child's sex we didn't want to know it. Girl or boy—we didn't want to know.

The heart was pumping. The floating form was still. Across the chest and the skull there were pale areas like clouds. "The fetus is unquestionably edemic," the doctor said, pointing to the paleness that would otherwise have seemed ordinary to us.

"We've decided to abort it."

"Yes, Dr. Barrie has explained the situation."

Awakening around three A.M. from my drugged sleep, I noticed a new pain, a brief twinge inside my abdomen, wrapped in the other, constant pain. It hurt for a few seconds, then went away. After the night nurse helped me to the toilet and back to bed and gave me my scheduled pill for pain, I lay still on my left side and tried to sink into sleep.

The twinge shot horizontally across my swollen belly again and I wondered what it meant.

CHAPTER 3

BIRTH

I opened my eyes. Buried inside my bunker of pillows, I shifted slowly from my left side to my back, trying not to worsen the thick ache in my head and the burning in my abdomen. My left knee felt numb from the nightlong pressure of my right leg. The sheets were damp with sweat.

A nurse was standing by the window, a short, square figure in the gray light filtering through the blinds. "There now," she said with satisfaction, turning the window knob until the light filled the room.

"Not so much, please, just halfway."

"We've got ourselves another dreary day, I'm afraid." She raised her pudgy arm, readjusting the blinds. She had a busy, officious manner and was older than the other nurses; gray-haired except for a few brown streaks. "How about a shower? I'll help you."

I boosted myself into a sitting position, remembering to rely on my hands for support instead of my elbows, which had turned purple from repeated rubbing against the sheets.

"Easy does it," the nurse cautioned, as I sat on the edge of the bed, gathering my nerve to stand up. I leaned heavily on her as she inched toward the bathroom with me, her right arm encircling my waist, her left hand clasping my left arm. As I sat on the toilet, I could hear her bustling around the bed, stripping the linen.

I gripped the steel bar in the shower stall to steady myself and turned on the water. "Let me help you," the nurse said, opening the door.

"I'm all right, as long as I know you're out there." I didn't want her washing me like a child. Closing the door halfway, I let the johnny drop to the floor and stepped into the stall, clenching the bar with both hands. The spray of water fell on my swollen breasts and rounded belly, and for a while I just stood there leaning hard on the bar, staring at my body.

Back in bed, the clean sheets, the hot bowl of oatmeal on my bed table, the fresh johnny—I accepted these hospital comforts gratefully.

The nurse raised the steel bars on the right side of the bed. "Hoist yourself up with these when you want to sit up. It's easier than the way you're doing it."

For the second time that morning, I felt the twinge, like an electric arc shooting across my other pain. "I've had these twinges all night, on and off. Could they possibly be contractions?"

"Do you have a discharge?"

"No."

"Well, I don't think it's contractions then; maybe it's your fibroid."

"I don't think so, this is different from the fibroid pain."

"Well, you tell your doctor about it, dear, when he comes."

Dr. Lamont entered the room a few minutes after Dean and sat down in the chair by my bed. He looked tired. Dean was tidying my bed table, removing the messy breakfast tray and a clump of used tissues, neatly arranging my provisions for the morning: a cup of ice water with a flexible straw, a pitcher of ice water for refills, the morning paper he had brought, and the meal-order sheet for lunch and dinner laid on top of the newspaper with a pencil. Filling out the meal sheet was a hospital ritual I liked; I recall my pleasure in it coming as much from the sense of choice and control it gave me as from the anticipation of the food.

When I told Dr. Lamont about my twinges, he leaned forward, his hands pressing against his knees, his tie dangling, and he asked me questions: Exactly what do they feel like? How frequently do they come? When did they start? When was the last one? "I want to do an internal," he said. "I think your guess is right, I think you're having contractions." It only took a few seconds for him to measure me inside, measure the opening, the way I had always heard of doctors doing before a woman has her baby, when she thinks the time is coming. "There's no question about it, you're having contractions. I have a job for you, Dean. Write down the time each one occurs. Just keep a list for me. All day. I'll be back late this afternoon."

"I'm scared." I didn't want him to go. "I don't know what to do." The childbirth classes, the tour of the labor and delivery rooms, the planning. "We never learned about this."

"You won't be ready to deliver until tonight some time. Dr. Barrie will be here then. It's really best this way, you know. Better than having to induce it. We'll give you a caudal to numb your lower body when the time gets closer. In the meantime, when the contractions come, just take slow, deep breaths. Dean, you can help her with this by reminding her to concentrate on the breathing and to breathe deeply."

Dean and I practiced on the next twinge, while Dr. Lamont looked on. Dean's voice was confident, soothing. I remember marveling at the unselfconscious way he took on the job, as though he was an old hand at it. "Okay, now, Marion, breathe in slowly, deep breath. Now out, slowly, that's it, slowly." The breathing helped. The clenching pain passed more easily.

"One thing you both need to consider," Dr. Lamont said, "it would be wise for you to see your child."

"See our child!" I was dumbfounded. So was Dean. "We couldn't bear it. We don't even want to know the sex. The less we know the better."

Dr. Lamont's cow eyes looked at me intently, and then at Dean. "It's easy to understand why you feel that way."

For a minute or two, the three of us sit in silence. Images of newborn babies form in my mind. I see them as snapshots, the kind fathers take when the nurse holds up the baby at the nursery window. I see each child two-dimensionally, angry red fists clenched forever inside a shiny white paper border.

"It's easy to understand," Dr. Lamont repeated, "but our experience with other couples tells us that you'll be better off afterwards if you've seen your child. If you don't see the child, you're likely to regret it when it's too late. It will be important for you to know that your child was born and was not able to live, but wasn't monstrous in any way. You're going to need a picture in your mind, so you don't go around imagining things that aren't true. Trust me in this. Think about it. Talk together about it. You can let me know later."

"Do you think Dr. Barrie would agree with you?"

"Oh, no question. She would want you to see the baby."

When Dr. Lamont left, Dean closed the door and came to stand beside the bed. He looked down at me for a while, and then, wheeling the bed table out of the way, he leaned over me and we hugged each other tightly.

It had all been unthinkable a week before—still seemed unthinkable. Loving each other, loving our child, loving ourselves, we had to bend all our love now toward helping me deliver our child dead.

All afternoon my contractions came at intervals of

five to fifteen minutes, and Dean wrote down the times in a long column under the heading: Sat. cramps. I guess he must have been thinking there might be another list for Sunday.

I ate well at lunchtime, anticipating that if all went as the doctor predicted I would have no dinner. Alongside his tidy column of cramp times—2:25 PM, 2:30 PM, 2:36 PM—Dean kept a list of what I ate, as the doctor had asked him to. Lunch-Sat., he wrote in his neat handwriting. And under that, in a column, he listed: 1/2 fruit cup, 1/2 cottage cheese, 1/3 yogurt, 1/3 tapioca, 1 bowl onion soup, 1 cup orange juice with Metamucil. In spite of the pain I was in, and in spite of the drugs, which made me constipated, nauseated, headachy, dizzy, mentally fuzzy, I was hungry—like any pregnant woman.

Shortly after four o'clock, Dr. Lamont returned and looked at Dean's lists and then measured the dilation of my cervix. The baby, he said, would be delivered that night. He instructed me again not to eat dinner, asked Dean to continue recording my contractions, and explained that the anesthesiologist would be in to talk to me.

"Does Dr. Barrie know what's happening?" I asked.

"I've spoken to her, so you needn't worry. She'll be here for the delivery."

Dr. Lamont paused. "Did you discuss what we talked about? Seeing the baby?"

"Yes," I said, shaken now in my conviction, so automatic and unquestioned before, that this should be a faceless, sexless child. Dean and I had agreed that we should be guided by Dr. Lamont and Dr. Barrie. "We'll follow your advice."

It was 6:35 when Dean made the last entry in his list. A few minutes later an orderly arrived with a stretcher—a sort of table on wheels—to take me to the delivery room. With Dean walking near, behind me, the orderly maneuvered me slowly yet dizzyingly down the corridor. Corridors and more corridors. The cavernous elevator. Corridors lower down, in a basement or subbasement, where a hospital weight of sickness and strange routines pressed down from above. I was feverish, and I could feel myself sweating into my hospital johnny under the two blankets draped over me. Yet I felt chilled and pulled the blankets up around my neck.

The delivery room looked ordinary. I don't know exactly what I expected, but I assumed the room would look like a room set up for the delivery of babies. It didn't.

There was an inhospitable-looking operating table at the far end of the room, well away from the door; it had a thin pad on it, covered with a sheet.

The delivery room nurse introduced herself and removed my blankets. There was no hesitancy about her; "let's get on with this" her motions seemed to say. I warned her—in the strange, slow, drunk-sounding speech I had been using for days—about my fever and my chills and my pain and my almost uncontrollable need to pee. She and Dean helped me move into a sitting position on the stretcher and then helped me stand up and inch my way into the bathroom.

When I came out of the bathroom, the stretcher was gone, and Dr. Lamont was standing in the empty middle of the room, dressed in a loose-fitting drab green gown, talking to Dr. Cary, the anesthesiologist whom I had already met.

"Is the pain from the fibroid worse?" Dr. Lamont asked. I nodded.

Dean and the nurse helped me up onto the table, sitting me down on the edge of it. My knees automatically spread wide, making my hospital johnny into a flimsy tent over my big belly. I put one hand behind me for balance, and with the nurse's arm around my back, lowered my upper body to the table while Dean lifted my legs and moved them onto the table, covering them and my belly with one of the hospital blankets.

I was shivering. "Aren't you cold, Deanie?"

Dean looked at me indulgently and shook his head. I was astonished that he wasn't cold.

The nurse spread two more blankets over me. Apologetically, Dr. Lamont lifted the sheet and blankets to my knees. He managed to examine me without making me move down on the table. When he was through, I asked for a pillow to place under my right knee, and the nurse put one there, but still each second seemed more painful than the one before.

I had to pee again. The nurse offered a bed pan but I was incapable of holding myself over it. "I'd better just get up again," I said, but she continued to offer the pan, suggesting I stay where I was. I knew I couldn't use it, couldn't hold my buttocks even half an inch above the table. I was almost crying. "If someone doesn't help me down, I'm going to go right on the table."

"Help her down," Dr. Lamont snapped. "It will hurt her more to use the pan." The nurse stepped back as he came forward. He put an arm behind my back. "Easy now," he coached me. "Swing her legs around," he told the nurse.

"I'm sorry, I'm sorry," I kept apologizing.

Once I was resettled on the table, eased into position and covered with the blankets as before, the doctor told me Dean would wait outside while the anesthesiologist administered the caudal. I felt panicky about Dean not staying in the room, but he kissed me and whispered into my ear, "Hey, wipe off those furrows, I'll be right outside."

Dean told me later that he did his waiting in a crowded little room set aside for expectant fathers. I can imagine it, littered with old magazines and half-filled styrofoam coffee cups. A stuffy, depressing room for Dean, but not for the other men: the one excitedly jabbing his arms into the sleeves of a green hospital robe—"My wife's having a Caesarian"—or the one nervously chewing his thumbnails. "They wanted me out while they gave her the epidural. It's a girl. We know already. How about you?"

"Do I have to have an IV?" I asked the nurse.

"We want it, yes, in case you need any blood, but we don't anticipate that you will." I had never had an IV before, and I shrank from it as one more assault on my body and on my normal sense of control, already reduced nearly to extinction. The nurse inserted the needle neatly and quickly into the vein at my left wrist and taped it in place with an expert's ease. She looked down at me, her eyes very blue; they looked smooth, like the blue tiles above the sink in the wall facing me.

"Dr. Cary is going to insert the needle in your spine." The nurse helped me sit up and lean forward, enabling Dr. Cary, who stood behind me to my right, to open the back of my johnny and press around my spine with his fingertips. The pain was sudden, intense, sickening, stabbing my back. I gasped and moaned.

"All right?" Dr. Cary asked from behind me.

"Yes, I guess so." I calmed myself with the thought that the worst he could do to me was over.

"Now we just get the drug going through this tube," he said.

"Can I lie down?"

"Sure you can. It's all taped real well to your back, so don't worry about the needle moving, or the tube."

The nurse eased me down, and Dr. Cary moved around to my right side. He was tall and thin, and he had pasty, concave cheeks. But his face was gentle.

"Now, when the drug begins to flow, you'll feel a little pain."

"Bad pain?" I screwed my head to the right to see the bag of clear fluid hanging on the steel pole sticking out of the head of the table.

"Not too bad."

But it *was* bad. I was screaming. There was an explosion inside my right leg—glasslike splinters shooting from my hip to the tip of my foot. "My leg! My leg! My leg!" It would be ripped to shreds. Splattered everywhere.

The nurse's blue eyes stared steadily at me, and she stood motionless, leaning slightly towards me. "Are . . . you . . . sure . . . it . . . still . . . hurts?" She dragged out the words, like writing in the sky. I stared back at her, not screaming now, and concentrated my thoughts on her question. Does it still hurt? *My leg, does it still hurt?* And then I realized the pain was gone.

I must have fallen asleep soon after that, drifted away from the flat, indifferent surfaces of the room. For the first time in almost a week, I slept deeply. The caudal, numbing my body from the waist down, shut off the pain in my abdomen. I didn't notice this happen, didn't give it any thought. It was like the shutting off of a maddening siren; silence returns, frustration subsides, and the moment of change passes undetected. Not until much later, when the caudal wore off, exposing me again to the pain of the fibroid, did I realize what a respite I had had.

I felt a hand touch my cheek, grazing it gently. "Froggo, Froggo, try to wake up, it's almost time. You're doing well." I forced myself to open my eyes. Dean leaned over me and kissed my forehead. Dr. Lamont was standing beside him.

"I'm thirsty."

"I can't let you have any water," Dr. Lamont said, "but I'll moisten a washcloth for you and you can suck on it."

The damp cloth barely wet my mouth, and the feel and taste of the swollen threads between my teeth was repellant.

"I'm sorry, I wish I could do better for you, but I can't."

"Is Dr. Barrie here?"

"She's going to be here in a few minutes. Dean will stay with you now. I have to leave you, but you'll be okay."

"As long as you know Dr. Barrie is coming."

"She is. You needn't worry."

I grabbed the fingers of Dr. Lamont's hand in mine and pressed them firmly. "Thank you."

He smiled sadly, his lips drawn inward, his wide forehead creased, and he returned the pressure of my hand with a tight squeeze. He understood my gratitude.

I wasn't thinking then that I wouldn't see him again; but I haven't—except as a stranger, from a distance.

Dean sat down wearily on a straight-backed chair to my left, a few feet from the table I lay on. The back of his head touched a beige curtain that had been drawn parallel to the table during my sleep. I could no longer see the door or the large empty portion of the room. The idea, I suppose, was to increase my sense of privacy and protection. I was glad the curtain was there. It cut off the rest of reality, leaving me with the small part that mattered—me, and Dean, the table I lay on, and, when they arrived, Dr. Barrie and the nurse. And my belly, like an offering.

In the narrow space defined by the curtain and the three walls, the large, plain-faced clock high on the wall facing me was the only adornment, not counting the metal sink, and the cabinets above and beneath it. I stared at the clock, at the way the minute hand jumped nervously from minute line to minute line. I noticed the time, paid considerable attention to it, in fact. But later I couldn't recall how long I lay there or what time my child was born. "Before midnight or after?" I asked Dean.

"Before," he told me. So the birthdate was Saturday, May 28, and the time, Dean tells me, was about eleven-thirty. My hard labor—the part Dr. Barrie helped me through—the final pushing of the baby out into the world—took about an hour.

It was about ten-thirty, then, when Dr. Barrie came in, accompanied by the delivery nurse, and sat down on a low stool at the foot of the table. I kept complaining of the cold. The nurse arranged my blankets so the doctor could see what she needed to, while I was covered as much as possible. I could see nothing of what was happening between my legs. Dean, I knew, was watching for me.

"Squeeze down hard," Dr. Barrie said. "Good, real hard, like when you're moving your bowels." I strained with every muscle in my legs and thighs and buttocks and belly; and in the swollen tunnel made for bringing my babies into the world. Straining and straining to do it right, to have it over. "Good, very, very, good." Dr. Barrie's voice soothed and encouraged me. "Such a good job, it's almost over now, almost over. . . ."

"Squeeze my hand," said the nurse. I did. It helped. I gripped her hand with a strength that surprised me and pushed down on the table with my lower body as though trying to turn myself inside out.

"There! There!" Dr. Barrie said. And then, "Very good, very good . . . relax now, it's over." The nurse helped me move back up towards the top of the table and extend my legs, a pillow propped under my knees, the blankets covering my legs again. I lay with my eyes closed. I heard water running in the sink.

Dr. Barrie spoke to me, her voice by the table, at my right side. "I'm going to raise you a little now." She and the nurse put their arms around me and helped me into a sitting position, adjusting the table to support my back. I kept my eyes closed, wanting only to sleep, to fall away from the room into oblivion. "I'm going to let you hold the baby now," the doctor told me firmly, calmly. I shook my head back and forth, weeping. "I can't . . . I can't . . . I can't . . . ."

"This is important for you, Marion. I'll help you, I'll help you. I'm right here." And I felt a weight being placed in my arms, and the doctor leaning intently

over me. "Open your eyes, Marion, it's okay to look
. . . it's a little girl."

Oh, God, not a little girl, not a little girl. I was sobbing,
holding the child, still refusing to see. *Not a girl, not a
girl.*

I felt as though I would be stuck in that moment
forever, unable, as in a dream, to perform the one act
required of me. Had I indeed been dreaming, I would
have awakened then.

"Have you seen her?" I finally asked Dean, forcing
myself somehow to open my eyes and look at him
through my tears. He was sunk into the chair against
the curtain, and like everything in the room, he seemed
vividly present and yet at the same time physically
insubstantial, illusory, about to blur and fade.

"Yes. I saw her come out of you."

"I can't bear to look, Deanie."

"You can . . . you can. Go ahead . . . go ahead and
look."

I turned from Dean to look at the doctor, then followed her gaze downward, slowly, as though fighting
a physical paralysis, until I saw what I held. The doctor
gently pulled the pale pink blanket away from the face
and the body, until I could see the naked infant limbs,
the tiny girlish crotch, the expressionless, heavy-lidded
face. "It's a pretty little girl," said Dr. Barrie, touching
the flesh that was not pretty but oddly liver colored.
"You can see the swelling," Dr. Barrie instructed, her
voice quiet, assured. She touched the baby's temple
where it was swollen and pocked like a sponge. The
chest and one of the arms and one of the legs were
spongelike too. "You can touch her," Dr. Barrie said to
me, guiding the tips of my fingers down the soft,
unpocked flesh of the left arm. My tears were falling
on the small, dark body.

And then the doctor swaddled the baby again and
lifted her up and carried her to Dean. "Would you like
to hold her?"

Dean looked at me, his eyes brimming with tears. I nodded at him, unable to speak. Go ahead, my eyes told him, hold her, be brave. When the doctor placed the baby in his arms and pulled back the blanket from the lifeless flesh, Dean bowed his head and sobbed. I'd heard him cry before, and I've heard him since. But never like that—desperate, high-pitched explosions of grief and love.

CHAPTER 4

LOSS

1

Dean tells me I fell asleep soon after the doctor took the baby from his arms.

I wasn't aware who carried the baby from the room, or at what moment precisely, or how she was held—embraced like a sleeping child, or carried in some kind of sack or box. Her presence in that room was ghastly, nightmarish. I gladly let her dissolve into the space past the end of the table, where the doctor and the nurse moved like shadows.

Today I can't help trying to imagine her being carried from the room, and I wish I could pull her back, prevent her from being spirited away. I wish I could hold her in the daylight, see her, smell her, feel her, knowing what I know now. I would still be terrified, but I would have the chance for a longer, more conscious good-bye.

That night, though, I gratefully sank into a deep sleep, benefited by the drugs still numbing my lower body, and the catheter that, without my being conscious of it, was functioning for me. Dean "watched over me," as he explained it to me later, from his chair between the curtain and the table. I can imagine him sitting there, the lights shut off in the room, his eyes becoming accustomed to the dark; light from the hall seeping weakly under the door and under the curtain; the clock on the wall clicking faintly every sixty seconds, the minute hand jumping forward—click, jump, click, jump. I can imagine him sitting there, unable to stop seeing the baby, stop feeling her weight against his arms; and unable to stop sitting there, needing to be near me.

Someone was touching my arm, prodding me awake. "Marion, Marion." I opened my eyes and saw the nurse and Dean and the curtain and the clock. It was nearly two A.M. The room was in half-light. I heard a voice in the hall; the door was open. For seconds, just a few seconds, it was all a puzzle, the pieces threatening to come together yet still separate. And then I remembered how it all fit: emptiness—nothing—where something loved had been.

The abdominal pain was there again too, the son-of-a-bitch pain was still there. "Why did you wake me?" I asked the nurse, my words like small claws scratching the air.

"I'm going to remove the needles, and then we'll get you back upstairs."

"It hurts again. I need a pill, and I need to eat something, I'm starving."

"I'll get you a Tylox."

"No, just water, please, I want the pill in my room. I want to be in my room." I started crying.

Dean took my hand and stroked my fingers with his fingertips. "Maybe you should take the pill now, it will help."

"No, just water, I want the pill in my room." I remember feeling irrationally, childishly distrustful of the nurse, afraid she would give me the wrong medication, and I remember thinking of my hospital room as truly mine, a haven I wanted to flee to.

The nurse gave me a cup of ice water, and Dean

helped me raise my head to drink. My head was aching, and my throat was so parched it felt swollen and the crying hurt. The nurse untaped my wrist where the needle was, and I looked away while she slipped the needle from my vein. "Hold this here for a few minutes," she said, pressing a gauze patch against my wrist.

"Now the back." Dean helped me sit up and lean forward, and I felt the tape rip away from my skin; then a brief, sickening pain as the needle left my spine.

"Can I lie on it? Won't it hurt?"

"Go ahead and lie down, you'll be fine."

I continued to lean forward, putting painful pressure on the fibroid.

"Really, you'll be all right, lean back." Dean and the nurse supported my weight as I lay slowly down against the table, and they pulled the blankets up over my belly and chest.

"You're right, it's okay." The nurse looked at me, pleased. Then she left the room.

Dean kissed me on the forehead and on the lips, and in the corners of my eyes, where tears were leaking. "Here, use these," he said, bringing me a box of tissues from the cabinet beneath the sink.

"Why don't they go ahead and move me to my room?"

"This table has to stay here, she's getting another one and someone to move you. She'll be back soon."

"You can move me."

"They won't let me, I asked them."

"Well, why doesn't she move me?"

"She can't leave, she's the only one on duty."

"Well, why the hell did she wake me?"

"She's doing her best, Froggo."

"It's so late. Are you going to stay with me?"

"Yes, don't worry, I'm not leaving."

Dean slumped in his chair like a stuffed Halloween effigy, his shoulders pulled forward, his head sagging against his chest. I wanted to stroke the top of his head and wished he could lie down beside me. "You're exhausted."

"Yes, I am."

The room was eerily quiet, and no sound came from the hall. "Where the hell is she?"

Dean got up and kissed me again. "I'll go check."

"Don't go far." He disappeared around the curtain.

The intercom went off in the hall. "Doct," then nothing, the message unfinished. I heard footsteps coming toward my door; a shuffling, slippered sound, continuing past, slowly fading to a faint shhh, then silence. It was two-fifteen. I watched the clock: click, jump, click, jump. The pain burned so fiercely I could scarcely believe I had just spent several hours free of it. Why did they wake me, I kept thinking, why did they wake me into this pain?

"Get meeeeee out of heeeeere!" My screaming tore through the room and out into the empty corridor like a flock of mad jays flapping and screeching.

The eerie quiet formed again for an instant; footsteps ran through it. Dean and the nurse were standing beside me.

"What happened? What happened?"

"Get meeeeee out of heeeeere!"

Astonishment and panic gave the nurse's eyes a wild, trapped look. She moved me just as I was—the table, the layers of blankets, the box of tissues I was holding. The way she rushed me from the room, it might have been on fire.

As the nurse helped Dean maneuver me off the table into a sitting position on my bed, I realized for the first time that the table and my hospital johnny were soaked with blood.

"I have to hand it to you," said Dean, chuckling, as soon as the nurse had gone, "you sure scared the hell out of us. I bet they heard you screaming out on

Brookline Avenue. You should have seen that nurse running down the corridor."

Dean helped me into the bathroom, and I put on a clean johnny and a pair of underpants, and from the shelf beside the toilet I took a sanitary pad for the blood. Somehow I hadn't expected this blood, hadn't anticipated it at all. Startling. Infuriating. What should have been a joyful bloodletting—the cathartic end of pregnancy, the undamming of new life—was instead the blood of death.

When I looked myself in the eye in the bathroom mirror, I expected to see more a mask than a face— something remote, despairing, old. Of the incongruities of that night, one of the oddest was my face in the mirror: I was still me. I think what surprised me most was to see my look returned.

When I came out of the bathroom, Tina was in the room placing a pitcher of ice water on my table and talking to Dean. The instant she looked at me, I started to cry. "I lost my baby, Tina, I lost my baby."

"I know, I know," she said, coming to me and putting her thin arms around me, hugging me. "I know, I know." She helped me settle into bed, arranging the bank of pillows and makeshift pillows so I could sit up. "Now," she said, when I had swallowed the Tylox capsule she gave me, "Dean tells me you're starved. What would you like?"

Dean had left the room and was returning with two pillows and as many of the thermal blankets as he could hold. He piled everything on the windowsill and bent over to prepare a bed for himself on the floor between the window and my bed. "You poor thing, how will you sleep?" I asked.

"Don't worry, I'm so tired the floor will be fine. Can I shut off the light?"

The only light on in the room was the one midway up the wall behind the head of my bed. That was the light—not harshly bright, but strong enough to be reassuring—that I had come to like having on for a while at night before I fell asleep. I didn't need it, though, with Dean there. I pulled the string safety-pinned to my sheet and the light went out.

The room was dark except for the light coming from the hall. I had gotten into the habit of not letting the night nurse close the door until after I fell asleep. Even then, the light in the bathroom stayed on all night, a night-light of sorts, leaking into the room through the slit between the floor and the bottom of the bathroom door; just the faintest hint of light, because I was afraid of waking there in complete darkness.

"Will it be okay if the door is open?" I asked Dean. "Just until I eat something?"

"Sure. Good night." Dean leaned over to kiss me and I put my arms around his neck and held him against me.

"I love you."

"I love you, too."

Soon I could hear Dean's light snoring, a purring sound he makes only when he's exhausted.

Tina came in with the tray of food. She had poured a thin layer of milk on top of the Jell-O, the way I liked. "I'm glad you're on duty tonight," I told her.

"I am, too. I'll leave the door open until you're asleep."

"Thanks, good night."

I fed myself the Jell-O slowly, as though I was feeding an infant. The light from the hall fell weakly on the surfaces in the room—on the blankets covering Dean's sleeping form, on the picture of Charlie Brown, on the arrangements of flowers along the windowsill, on Dean's clothes thrown over the chair. I was glad Dean was snoring. We couldn't lie close enough to touch each other, but the soft sound was like a hand I could hold. Dean and I still had each other. We would abide, in spite of everything—in spite of the blood leaking out between my legs; in spite of the emptiness.

Finally I lowered the bed and closed my eyes.

*   *   *

In the morning, feeling Dean's kiss on my lips, and hearing his promise, faint and faraway, to return in the afternoon, I kept my eyes closed and retreated like a burrowing creature into the safety of sleep. Some terrible consciousness waited for me. I shrank from it.

It was to be that way every morning; now, every waking would be a reluctant waking, a waking into absence.

When my physical pain finally forced me awake, the room was depressingly dark. Only a pale settling of morning light seeped in around the blinds and through the drawn curtains. The flowers on the sill—the daisies my parents had sent, the lilies from my brother and his wife—looked trapped in the dull light. I loved the shapes of them, wanted to see sunlight shining on the petals and leaves, but I wanted, too, to smash the planters, one by one—slam them against the sill, or hurl them through the glass of the window.

There was a Band-Aid on my wrist where the needle had been. I ripped it off and gently touched the black and blue skin underneath.

My belly still formed a dome under the covers, as though an animal slept there, curled up, keeping me company. But the big belly was a fake now. The baby was gone—not sleeping near me, sucking and grasping the air, not floating in me either.

I put on the radio and happened to find something I recognized and liked: Brahms's Second Piano Concerto, the slow movement, slow and gentle as the rocking of a cradle or the lapping of lake water at a child's feet; sad, as though each note is a memory.

When Dr. Barrie came in to see me, the movement was just ending. I started to weep—quietly, involuntarily, not asking the doctor for help or sympathy, but as though crying and breathing were one function, impossible to untangle. "I'm sorry," I said. The concerto was still playing. I shut it off.

"Don't apologize. Of course you're crying." Dr. Barrie stood by my bed and asked me questions about how I was feeling—the amount of bleeding, the degree of pain in the fibroid, my ability to sleep. And she wanted to know about Dean. When had he left the hospital? When would he be back? Did he have any friends he could stay with for a night or two?

"I heard you created quite a stir downstairs last night." Dr. Barrie was laughing.

"That's what Dean tells me. I didn't really mean to scream that loud."

"Well, I don't blame you, you wanted to get out of that room. That was a bad place for you." She paused. "Your flowers are pretty. Can I open the curtains for you?"

"I'd like that."

"There are a few things I need to discuss with you." She sat in the chair by my bed. I had never noticed her so made-up before; her pale skin was pinker than usual, and blue shadow darkened her eyelids. Heavily powdered, her face had a vagueness that made her seem vulnerable, hinting of her life away from patients and deliveries. "We'll need permission from you and Dean to perform an autopsy. We really ought to, on the chance that we might learn something."

"I thought this was just a fluke, just bad luck."

"Well, yes, that's what we believe, but an autopsy would be wise."

"I'll mention it to Dean. I can't see any objection myself and I doubt that he'll have any."

I realized suddenly how distressed I was at the prospect of not seeing Dr. Barrie again after I left the hospital. I still needed her, yet she was, after all, my obstetrician; what claim would I have to her time, with the baby gone?

What I feared then, and what I continued to fear in the months to come, was that the process Dean and I had begun would come to an end—an end defined only by loss. Rationally or not, when I contemplated no longer seeing Dr. Barrie, I felt abandoned, and my hope for a second pregnancy shriveled. If I were to believe that my childbearing had not come to a permanent end, I needed Dr. Barrie to help me believe.

"I don't know how to say this . . . I'm scared about not seeing you anymore."

"Not seeing me?"

"Yes, when I go home."

Dr. Barrie laughed. She must have been happy to have at least one point on which she could tell me what I wanted to hear. "Oh, we'll be seeing plenty of each other, don't you worry about that. I'm not leaving you alone. Even if you wanted me to. For one thing, we have your fibroid to deal with. We have a long way to go together yet."

Oddly, it hadn't occurred to me that the fibroid problem would remain Dr. Barrie's concern. Reluctantly, I asked her, "What about the fibroid?"

"It should shrink a little in the next few months. I hope we can put off operating for six months or so. That will give you time to get your strength back and to ease your way into working again. If the pain decreases in the next few days, which it should, we'll get you out of here."

"Did the fibroid start to hurt because the baby was dying?"

"Yes, in hindsight, I do think that is why the pain began."

"It was a kind of alarm."

"You could say so, yes."

"It's funny, you know, I don't want to leave, I don't want to go home."

"That doesn't surprise me really, but it will be good for you to go home. You could use some fresh air; it's not good to be sealed up in here so long. And I know Dean needs you at home."

"He does, you're right. But I'm afraid I'll just be a burden, so sick like this."

"Oh, I'm sure he'd rather have you home than here in the hospital. You won't be a burden, we'll see to that."

"The weather still isn't much like spring, is it?" The expanse of hospital roof stretching below the tower was a dull reddish color, darkened by days of rain and drizzle, and blotched with puddles. In the distance, on the topmost level of the parking lot, five cars, toy-sized from my perspective, waited in the gray light of the morning, looking abandoned, like props on an empty stage.

"The weatherman is predicting a sunny week. When you get home and you're feeling a little better, you can sit outside. I'm sure the sun will be out by then, and it will do you good."

But I was thinking that I didn't want to go outside, didn't want to sit in the sun. Without the prospect of my growing big, of planning and preparing for motherhood, I would be like my neighbor's tree that had remained bare last spring and summer. They hadn't cut it down, and it was still standing there, its skeleton of branches again insisting that winter had never ended.

"I'll be able to have children after the operation, won't I?" I asked the question that I had told myself not to ask yet.

"I'm optimistic. There's a surgeon here at Brigham and Women's whom I'm going to talk to about performing the surgery with me. She's an expert at these operations, and I know she'll do all she can to leave as much of your uterus intact as possible. You see, everything depends on how deep the fibroid is lodged in the uterine wall and on precisely how it's positioned. With such a large tumor, the amount of uterine tissue we cut away can impair your ability to carry a child. We also worry about your tubes becoming scarred, and about bleeding; if cutting away the tumor causes a dangerous amount of bleeding, we have to remove the uterus. Those are unlikely outcomes though, Marion, they really are. In about 90 percent of these operations, the patient goes on to bear a child. I'm hoping to get you all fixed up for a second try."

"Part of me can't bear the thought of not trying again, and part of me can't bear the thought of trying. What if . . ."

Dr. Barrie nodded. "I know. But think of it in a way that makes you feel good. Don't think of it as an ordeal, because you're still in the middle of this one, and you've got to allow yourself time to heal. When you're stronger, and when the operation is behind you, you'll find the courage to try again, I know you will. It won't seem as difficult then as it does now." She stood up, pressing her hands against her skirt, smoothing it. Her arms and legs were fleshed out, not bony at the wrists and ankles like mine, and it always struck me, when I happened to notice, that her breasts would have seemed voluptuous on someone else. There was an endearing confusion to Dr. Barrie's appearance; her womanliness was at odds with her wide, inquiring eyes and her straight, slightly scraggly hair that made it so easy to picture her as a girl.

"I have a patient in labor now, but I'll be back this evening." It never ceased to amaze me how she moved with such calm matter-of-factness from one grave responsibility to another.

As she left the room, I struggled to keep my thoughts on her kindness, but it was impossible to stifle my resentment at her mentioning that other patient. Hadn't she known how jealous it would make me feel? That other woman would be someone without difficulties, no doubt, someone in the ordinary routine; and Dr. Barrie would be seated at the foot of the table, intent on the emerging infant, a healthy boy or girl.

I seemed to be wishing that woman anything but a healthy child. You never knew, it could happen, the child might be dead like mine, or might be born with some terrible problem. Yes, I had to admit, I was wishing it. This stranger out there, I wanted her to suffer too.

A nurse came in and reached for the blood pressure sleeve hanging on the wall behind me. I put my arm out obediently. "I think I'd like to be able to watch the television. Do you know what I have to do to get it switched on?"

"Just call the number up there." The nurse pointed to the television that had been staring blankly at me for five days. I hadn't noticed the writing on it before, in print large enough to be readable from the bed: FOR SERVICE, CALL EXTENSION 2748.

The serviceman knocked on my door—a sallow-skinned man with eyes like a spaniel's. He carried a metal box, and in his gray pants and work shirt (*Hospital Media Services, Inc.* was stitched above the breast pocket), he looked out of place, not medical. There was something unsettling about that, as if he were a dispensable part in an otherwise tightly designed machine.

"Paying now? Or should I have them bill you?" He reached up to the television and inserted a key into a lock I hadn't noticed.

"How much?"

"Two fifty a day."

"You can bill me, I guess. What if I want it off again? I really don't watch much television. I've been here five days without it."

"Patients love it. They all do. It helps them pass the time."

"Still, though, what if I want it off?"

"Just call us again, the same number as before," he said, and he left, perhaps offering a silent thanks that most patients weren't like me.

The remote control gadget elicited a loud *ka-chunk* from the television each time I pressed it, as the television jumped to the next channel. I hated the sound and hated the series of seven or eight *ka-chunks* I had to submit to before I could reach the "off" position.

The first show I tuned to was an *All in the Family* rerun. Gloria was pregnant and Edith was crocheting a blanket for the baby-to-be. My ex-mother-in-law had crocheted a blanket for my baby, the color of daisies and green moths; I might never get to use it. I hated Gloria and Edith. I pressed the control.

My head ached and my eyes were tired, but I lay there staring upward trying to concentrate. "Look Ma, no cavities," yelled a freckled-faced girl with blond braids; she slammed a pile of schoolbooks onto a kitchen table and tilted her head back, mouth open. She looked like an overgrown young robin waiting for a worm. I hated her, and I hated the mother, who looked about my age. She probably has other kids, too, I thought, what does she know. *Ka-chunk* again. Next, an ad for "Huggies, the disposable diaper that . . ." The world was nothing but parents and children, children and parents. *Ka-chunk, ka-chunk, ka-chunk, ka-chunk.*

The next day I called the television service and the same man came to shut off the brown box. "You surprise me, lady, you surprise me. Most patients, they wouldn't be without it." He held his key aloft and fitted it into the lock. I said nothing, smiling insincerely until he left the room, carrying his little metal box of money and keys.

If only he could have taken with him the murky, incapacitated screen. Of all the fixtures in the room, it was the most offensive to my efforts and Dean's to make the room mine. I wanted every object justified in terms of utility or homeyness or beauty. The television failed every test. It depressed and antagonized me.

Nothing I perceived was neutral. There were two categories of people and things: those that helped, and those that hurt.

Tuesday, the day before I went home, a hospital social worker came to see me, offering me several typed pages of information. Urging me to read them. The heading on the first page: "A Funeral For Your Baby." Another heading, simply: "Grief."

"Cremation is offered by the hospital without cost," the social worker explained. "You and your husband should discuss whether you want the hospital to handle everything for you or whether you wish to have a funeral. If possible, let us know before you leave; but if you need more time, you can mail in the form." She handed me a form entitled CONSENT FOR DISPOSITION OF FETAL REMAINS. It read as follows:

> Under the Massachusetts Law, it is the responsibility of the Boston Hospital for Women to inform its patients of their rights concerning burial of a stillbirth. In the event of a stillbirth which occurs on or following twenty weeks of pregnancy or a weight of 350 grams or more, the parent(s) may choose to bury, cremate, or entomb the fetal remains.
>
> For those parents needing information concerning burial, cremation and entombing the Admitting Office will recommend the services of a local undertaker. Please call 732-4005.

PLEASE INDICATE YOUR CHOICE:

_____ I wish to assume the responsibility for the disposition of the fetus.

_____ I do not wish to assume the responsibility for disposition of the fetus and release the remains to the hospital for disposition in a

manner consistent with provisions of Chapter 598 of the Massachusetts Laws.

Patient Signature
<hr>

<hr>
Date

2

On Wednesday, June 1, after eight nights in the
hospital, I sat in a wheelchair in the hospital lobby,
looking through the glass doors, watching for Dean's
car. "That's him," I said, and the orderly wheeled me
onto the rubber ramp, through the automatic doors
and out into the fresh air. It was chilly in the shade of
the cement canopy that sheltered the driveway, but the
sunny street beyond promised a warm day; it felt odd
to be so close to that open, bright street.

"She's going to lie down back here," Dean said to
the orderly, lifting the hatch of the station wagon,
revealing a nest of sleeping bags, blankets and pillows.
The orderly helped Dean support me as I stood up in
front of the wheelchair and sat down on the back edge
of the wagon with my feet on the pavement and the
hatch door open over my head.

"That's a great idea. You've got quite a comfortable-
looking bed there." The orderly seemed genuinely impressed with Dean's handiwork. "You take good care
of yourself now," he told me, turning to reenter the
lobby.

I inched back into the wagon, wincing at the pain of
the fibroid, and lay down. Dean closed the hatch, and
we were moving, the cement and glass and steel of the
hospital looming over me, filling my view, disappearing. Tears formed that I had been fighting back all

morning. It was over. Our baby was gone. We were going home without her.

I was bedridden for nearly two weeks at home, sleeping most of the time, getting out of bed only to limp the short distance to the bathroom. The space I moved in seemed compressed, stifling, as it had in the hospital, my concentration and mobility limited by drugs and pain, the range of my thoughts limited by grief.

Any convalescent lives through those insular, inward-looking hours in bed with an acute sense of aloneness and vulnerability. For me this sense was overwhelming, fed as it was by two forces, my illness and my loss. I lay in bed confronting, every second of the day, the absence within my body—the presence of one heart where two had been. I had grown accustomed to taking care of the dependent being inside me; now I had only myself and Dean to think about. I was one again, and Dean and I were two again; the threesome we had gotten used to and made plans for was gone. Home from the hospital, I had to fit myself back into the world with a piece missing.

It was impossible not to compare my situation to what it would have been if I had just come home from the hospital with a newborn. I felt cheated, imagining all the would-have-been details. And my body encouraged the comparison; my still-swollen belly and my swollen breasts knew that my child had been delivered but not that she had died. The intermittent fluttering I felt in my abdomen as my uterus began contracting was, so far as I could guess, no different from the twinges I would have felt after a live birth; and my breasts, veined, tender, looking like someone else's, had begun to fill with milk.

I loved and hated the sight of my breasts. All my longing seemed embodied there—my futile aching to nourish a new life. The tenderness would pass in a few days, but I didn't really want it to; I wanted the milk to be there, and a sucking mouth. What would it have been like, I wondered. Why should other women—those I pictured bent forward over an infant's fussing, tugging body—have that experience and not I?

Dean stayed home with me for several days. When he left the house to shop or to give himself a break from taking care of me, I was possessed by the fear that I couldn't survive his absence, that somehow I would lose even the little strength and lucidity I had. I was particularly afraid to maneuver my way into the bathroom alone; and, though I did get that far, I didn't dare continue down the hall and through the dining room into the kitchen for something to eat or drink.

I was afraid for Dean's welfare, too. Whenever he went out, I worried obsessively that some terrible accident would befall him. Who would care for me? Who would calm me when I woke up during the night? Who would share my sorrow? Now that bad luck had elected me out of hundreds, thousands, to lose my child, I had no faith that Dean, too, would not be taken from me. When he kissed me good-bye the morning he returned to work, I studied his face as though we would never see each other again. That became a habit with me every morning for a long time.

Once Dean returned to work, as Dr. Barrie encouraged him to do for his own well-being, the doctor took it upon herself to help me through the days, phoning me every few hours, telling me at each call when I could expect her to call again. She listened carefully to my descriptions of my pain, my dizziness, my weakness, and she reassured me and made suggestions about the level of my medication. If I was worried about needing her advice in the evening, she would promise to call me then too, and she never disappointed me. As nearly as was possible, she made herself a substitute for the professional nurses I no longer had. She called me before a delivery or after a delivery, or even from her home on her day off. Her singsongy "hi," sweet and clear, was always precisely the same, like the call of a bird, and it made me smile. She understood how much I needed her, and she didn't mind—indeed, insisted—that I lean on her.

She and I spent much of our time on the phone discussing the pills I was taking for pain. They had become an obsession with me. I was supposed to take no more than one or two of the Tylox capsules (a mixture of codeine and Tylenol) every three hours, continuing my hospital routine; but in the hospital the nurses had monitored the schedule, and I had needed only to pester them when they were slow bringing me a pill, while at home I had to keep track of the three-hour intervals myself, pushing my dulled powers of recall and concentration to the limit. I worried that I might take an extra pill, worsening the oppressive side effects, or might miss a pill, worsening my pain. I became frightened whenever I thought I had made a mistake, and I tried different mnemonic devices as protection.

In the middle of one night I woke up feverish and disoriented and became convinced that I had taken too much medication. In my panic, I had a kind of fit— violent, uncontrollable shaking and cramps—that I honestly thought I might not survive. Dean recalls me being so hysterical with fear that I was unable to instruct him how to help me.

After that, I put away the prescription medication and relied on ordinary Tylenol. Without the codeine, the fibroid burned badly, but at least it had detectably improved since the day I entered the hospital, enough to be bearable.

During those weeks of illness, always present, weightier than anything else I felt, was the sense of grief, of mourning. This made me grateful to have that quiet, private time in which to think—time away from well-meaning but misunderstanding friends and relatives and strangers. I chose my few visitors carefully.

Defining what it was Dean and I had lost proved difficult enough for the two of us. Small wonder, then, that most other people were lacking in understanding. A stillborn child defies one's usual ways of thinking about life and death: such a child has died but has never lived, has been born but has never breathed. And in my case the child had not even been carried to term, had never developed to the point of being capable of life.

Though I mourned the child I had lost, I was determined to replace her. When I fantasized about a second pregnancy, it was vital that the child be a girl, not a boy. And that girl was to be named Amelia, while the child I had lost would remain nameless. To that extent, at least, I believed that I could make up for what had happened to me.

Some people I spoke to seemed to think that what I needed was to find reason and fairness in what had happened. But just the suggestion that there was something benign about my loss made me want to scream or cry.

"I know how hard it is," Dean's mother was saying over the phone.

No you don't, I thought. You've got three kids. You never lost one.

". . . but it's God's will, we can't always understand His reasons."

Reasons? What reasons? What did reason and planning have to do with losing my child? What I had been through was the antithesis of reason, goodness, plan, purpose.

When sympathy and the defense of God were offered to me as part of the same package, it helped me to think of Rabbi Kushner. The social worker at the hospital had recommended his book and Dean had brought it home from the library: *When Bad Things*

Happen to Good People. The title gave me a group to belong to, good people unfairly afflicted. Rabbi Kushner was in this group himself; his little boy had been one of those children who age like an image on film running forward too fast, a tiny old man taunted by other kids, then *poof,* gone. Rabbi Kushner armed me to deal with the upbeat comments. He observed that I didn't have to smile and nod agreement when people said "It's God's will, it must be for the best." If it hurt me too much to keep my mouth shut, I could tell people I had a different opinion, I could explain that I didn't think there could be any sense to what had happened, didn't ever expect to see my tragedy as "for the best." I needed this kind of permission. So did Dean.

Speaking to anyone—face to face, or on the phone—was like going swimming with my brother when we were kids. You had to be on guard. Any minute you might be splashed or dunked or flipped backwards. You might even be held under long enough to make you scared. It was dangerous, unpredictable business.

Before I even left the hospital, I began to fear the misguided remarks; each one would wash away another piece of the little island Dean and I were standing on. Some of the phone calls I made before going home were intended as bulwarks against that erosion.

Of special concern to me was the couple who lived next door to us. They had been so warmhearted about the pregnancy; they were grandparents used to getting excited about babies, and they had given us the little stuffed toy chick we put in the baby's room. What if I got home and they asked me with knowing smiles how I was feeling or what names Dean and I had chosen? And what if Dean got home from the hospital one evening and ran into them with their cheerful assumptions?

When I made the preventative phone call from the hospital, I could hear my slurred, slow voice going into details about the birth and holding the baby. I wanted to stop but I couldn't. You're embarrassing her, something kept telling me on the edge of my brain. But I kept on.

"I'm sorry, real sorry," I finally let my neighbor say. "I'm glad you let us know." But she didn't sound glad.

At home, when I was finally able to lie outside on a lawn chair, I faced away from our neighbor's house and hoped she would ignore me. But she came over and greeted me, her voice flapping the air cheerfully like a flag on a sunny day. "Beauty of a day, isn't it?" She stood there, hands on hips, head tilted back, approvingly studying the cloudless sky.

I had placed my chair so I could look at my roses, fist-sized cutouts of color—white, yellow, pink, lavender. I liked to say their names to myself: Garden Party, Heirloom, Double Delight—a litany of luxuries. And I loved the way the colors hung there in the sun, beyond the tight package of my depression sealed to me like plastic wrapping.

"Are you feeling pretty good, now? You look a little tired."

I felt exposed and exhausted. I tried to think of something truthful I could bring myself to say. "I'm a little better, but it will take a while, and then I may need surgery. I have a fibroid tumor that's still very painful."

"Well, you get some sun. That and rest and you'll be thinking about trying again before you know it."

She made it sound so simple, just like waiting for the next bloom on the rosebush, nothing to it.

I went in the house and lay down and cried myself to sleep.

My impulse was to hide from people, to withdraw, and as a result, although the lawyers and secretaries I worked with had been kind, sending me flowers and cards, I dreaded returning to work and didn't do so for nearly two months. Dean, on the other hand, plunged rapidly back into his regular routine, and many of the people he worked with had no idea something had gone wrong in his life, that indeed he was mourning the loss of a daughter. Co-workers who had heard I was pregnant were still congratulating him on the "great news" or slapping him on the back with a "What's it gonna be, a girl or a boy?" Most of those who had heard about the stillbirth avoided the subject out of embarrassment or confusion. Or they said something unmindful of Dean. "Tell Marion I'm really sorry about her loss." Or, "I heard about Marion's loss. How is she doing?" Dean observed that there was no predicting who would say something witless and who would turn out to be gentle, knowing. He discovered that a few co-workers had had losses of their own, losses they rarely spoke of. Now, they offered their tragedies as gifts. Dean came home and told me their stories, and we felt a little less alone.

A few of our friends and relatives had had losses too. I wrote a letter to long-time friends of mine whose son had been stillborn the previous winter. They lived in England, but I felt a connection to them now that was like a physical pull across the space between us. Soon an answer arrived, an eight-page letter I read over and over and kept—and still keep—in the drawer by my bedside. "I received your letter this morning," Stella wrote. "I have phoned George at work and we are *so* terribly sorry for your loss. You are going through a terrible time, I know. I am grateful to you for writing to us. I understand now that however sorry people are, nobody can experience the hopeless, desolate feeling that one feels, except someone who has been through it. I remember one night ripping to pieces a cardigan I was making for the baby, and throwing things at the wall—anything! I threw a mirror across the room that night, but luckily for me it didn't smash. I don't need seven years' bad luck."

Another letter of sympathy arrived from an aunt who had heard about our loss through my mother. I had been somewhat out of touch with my Aunt Bernice for years, but now a correspondence began between us that gradually expanded to phone calls and visits. My aunt's first note to me, like those that followed, was short but filled with understanding. She knew from experience which words would help; knew what needed to be said, and what didn't. She knew, because one of her three young sons had died, about six years before, of leukemia.

I was grateful to my aunt for making the connection between her grief and mine. She might, it seemed to me, have dismissed my loss as insignificant compared to hers. Instead she recognized it as a bond between us.

One couple Dean had known since boyhood—people he thought of almost as second parents and whom I, too, had become fond of—paid us a surprise visit, staying long enough to share with us something we hadn't known: before adopting their daughter, they had lost two infants, a girl and a boy. Fran told me that eventually the pain would go away. From her, I could hear that without being angry. But even so, I was skeptical. Whatever might be true for her, I thought, my pain will never go away.

Dean and I were on different terms with the world than we had been before. One of the most dramatic effects of our loss was the new jealousy and hostility we lived with. Those feelings I had experienced watching television in the hospital persisted. And since the world is made up of children and parents and expectant parents and grandparents, it wasn't possible to watch television, or to read a newspaper or book, or to walk down a street, without feeling jealous and angry. When I was well enough to go shopping, I discovered that the supermarket was an especially difficult place for me; each time I saw a man or woman pushing a cart with an infant seated in it, I resented the very existence of parent and child and yet couldn't turn my eyes away. I remember one woman looking at me inquiringly, and my suddenly realizing, in embarrassment, that I had been standing still, leaning against my cart, staring at her infant in a kind of trance.

I disliked myself for my jealousy; it seemed so small-minded, and it cut me off from participating in other people's joy and from the pleasure I had always taken in children's faces and personalities. When I looked at children now there was no pleasure in it, only an angry longing and resentment; I wanted each child to transform into my lost child, or to disappear. When a healthy child was born to someone else, all I could think of was "that's not fair, why them and not me?" If I happened to be outside when my neighbor's daughter-in-law came to visit, getting bigger every week, expecting a baby just a month after mine had been due, I would rush inside. Later, I couldn't bear so much as a glimpse of her child, who had been carried in the womb at the same time as mine. The day of his birth, when I saw the banner my neighbor had draped across her garage—IT'S A BOY—all I could think of was that she should have considered me and not hung up that sign; I wanted to be protected, tiptoed-around.

For Dean, the great test of strength that summer was his secretary's pregnancy. She was expecting a child in August, and each day at work there she was for him to see, a little bigger, a little closer to becoming a mother. When she chatted at her desk with a friend about this or that aspect of her pregnancy, Dean closed his door so he wouldn't have to hear. When she complained about the weight she was gaining, Dean tried his best to be sympathetic.

Fortunately for Dean, his jealousy and anger chose their targets discriminatingly. While his secretary's pregnancy caused him suffering, he was much less apt than

I to become jealous of a television image or a stranger in a store. When we were in public and I saw a pregnant woman, I often leaned towards him and whispered, "I hate that woman, don't you?" "No I don't," he would say, "and you don't either. You hate what happened to you, but you don't hate her." For me, it always seemed impossible to make the distinction.

Sometimes Dean tried to comfort me with a favorite observation of his: "That woman may have her child," he would say, "but you have something she doesn't have." It was true, what he said. Though I found only the bitterest comfort in it, it was true. I had my experience of the coming together of birth and death, and though as a result I had become jealous, angry, even numb, I understood something I had never understood before about the preciousness of life. Sometimes I looked around me at other people and marveled that any of us were here at all. Certainly I marveled at my own existence and at Dean's.

CHAPTER 5

AUTOPSY

1

"Until we operate, we can never be certain, but I don't think it's too near your ovaries and it's not in the back of your uterus where it would be hard to get at."

Dr. Kagan, the specialist Dr. Barrie had recommended, probed me with her fingers, slowly, internally and pressing from the outside. Corroborating Dr. Barrie's judgment, and confirming my own instincts, she advised me not to get pregnant so long as the fibroid remained. She also warned me that if I didn't have the fibroid removed now, it would almost undoubtedly cause enough pain to have to be removed later anyway, in my forties or fifties; and there was a risk, a small risk, that the tumor, now benign, might become malignant, particularly during menopause. She spent a long time talking to me, explaining the risks of having the operation and the risks of not having it. Though she was optimistic that my surgery could be limited to what she called a myomectomy, an excision of the tumor, she emphasized that a hysterectomy might prove unavoidable.

"You're going to have to decide what to do. I have to admit, I wouldn't want to be in your position."

I had expected her simply to tell me what would be

done and when. But here I was, being asked to weigh the risks, to exercise control, though I felt I had none.

The pain of the fibroid had subsided by then into a mere hint of what it had been, but it was still a threat: if you push too far, it warned, you'll be sorry. I paid religious attention to it. I wore low-heeled shoes. I didn't ride my bike. I generally avoided driving the car, because the pain flared after I pressed the brake a few times; and when I had to drive I placed a pillow over my abdomen before I buckled the seat belt. In July, when Dean and I had gone to visit my parents, I had traveled lying down in the back of our station wagon, the same way I had come home from the hospital.

I was limited to wearing one of two old skirts with elastic waists—no jeans, no shorts; and I was beginning to wonder if my belly would ever return to its normal size. "It's as though you're still a few months pregnant," Dr. Barrie had told me two weeks earlier, at the beginning of August. "You'll never get those suits of yours back on until the tumor is gone. I don't think we should wait much longer for the operation, not with that tumor refusing to shrink."

"I'm scared," I said now to Dr. Kagan, embarrassed to find myself weeping.

"I know, I don't blame you."

"What would you do if you were in my place?"

"I'd have the operation. No question."

"You would?"

"Yes, I would."

"Thank you, I didn't really expect you to answer. I'll go ahead with it then, I'll do what you would do."

"Does it bother you that I'm pregnant?"

Oddly, I hadn't noticed. Now I saw the bigness I had been too preoccupied to see. It was there, under her white coat and what must have been a maternity dress. "No, it doesn't bother me."

Indeed, her pregnancy struck me as an advantage, the best possible assurance I could have that my sur-

geon would understand my fears, would understand
my asking her to be conservative, my asking her to cut
away as little of my body as she possibly could. "When
are you expecting?"

"The end of November."

"Do you have other children?"

"Yes, I'm fortunate. This will be my second."

"What if Dr. Kagan's baby kicks while she's operating?" I asked Dr. Barrie after we had scheduled my
surgery for September 23.

She laughed. "Babies don't kick that hard."

"Well, what about her belly getting in the way? Will
she be able to lean over? Will she be able to get close
enough?"

"She'll be perfectly comfortable, Marion, she'll adjust
the table to suit her needs. If there were any chance of
a problem, she wouldn't be operating."

When Dr. Kagan visited me in my hospital room two
days after the surgery, I was basking in the knowledge
that it had gone well. I still had my uterus; stitched
together, but able to hold a child.

Dr. Kagan was encouraging me to hope, to plan. She
wasn't even cautioning me that my tubes might be
scarred, as Dr. Barrie had cautioned me during her
visit. And she even thought I could deliver a child
vaginally again, rather than by Caesarian section; I was
surprised how much that mattered to me, how badly I
wanted another chance at doing the job myself.

"Discuss it with Dr. Barrie," she urged as she was
leaving. "See what she says—and have a good pregnancy." Those last five words, tossed to me so off-
handedly, I replayed over and over in my mind; I
received them as a prophecy.

I remained in the hospital for a week after my operation. The view from my window was a pleasant diver-

sion during that time, thoroughly unanticipated after the dismal tower and rooftop of my first stay. A restful scene, a composition primarily of color, order and pattern rather than activity: frame houses, variously painted, terraced on a hill of city streets; old trees bearing their splotches of green, red, yellow and orange above the angular roofs; a billboard—FLY DELTA—in iridescent violets and greens near the top of the hill; and at night, car lights, red and white, winking in and out of the dark beneath the spotlit sign. From where I lay in bed, I had a broad, safe perspective; faraway, the houses and cars kept their secrets, not burdening me with knowing the people in this landscape, the parents, the pregnant women. Here there were no mothers, no fathers, no infants, no children growing up.

My tumor had been cut away; but my grief was another matter. I was relieved at having the ordeal of surgery behind me—of course—and I was relieved, too, that the operation had been such a success, but the heaviness of mourning would not lift from me nor from Dean. When, out of habit, my old fantasy child tried to speak to me, I kept silent, learning to discourage, and finally, permanently, to stifle, that elfin voice. The depression, anger and jealousy that had followed the stillbirth remained, much more powerful than any stirrings of hope. On October 7—what once had been my due date—I was overwhelmed with emptiness, obsessed with what might have been. And again, as it had the first time, my convalescence encouraged bitter comparisons. Had I been recovering from a Caesarian delivery, I would have been having many of the same sensations—the numbness across my abdomen where the nerves were severed; the apprehensive holding in against coughs and laughs; the fascinated self-examination and protectiveness. (I was afraid even to lightly touch my scar. I might bleed, I might come apart.) How could I resist imagining myself in the circumstance of the new mother recovering from surgery? I could appreciate now how handicapped she would be in caring for her newborn—the fatigue she would feel, the difficulty holding and nursing her child. Mustering a sisterly sympathy for her legitimate complaints, I thought, too, how she would have missed something— the thrill of pushing a child into the world on her own. Yet how I envied her! Above all else, she would be feeling triumphant. Joyful.

It was around this time that Dean and I began to comprehend the perversity of mourning our child while refusing to fully recognize her, to think of or speak of her by name. Recognition and naming were, for us, intertwined. Denying our child a name, we were cutting away a crucial part of what she meant to us. Never legally required to name her (her death certificate had not required that she have a name, and she had no certificate of birth), we had referred to our child simply as "the baby" since the day of her death. Now, gradually—with help from a psychotherapist at our health center, a social worker whom we first visited at Dr. Barrie's suggestion shortly after the stillbirth and whom we continued visiting, on and off, for the next two and a half years—we came to admit that it was Amelia we had lost.

Until now, as though I had been introduced to someone and had turned away to stare out a window at someone else, I had been trying to imagine a child I might yet bear and call Amelia; but all along the name had been attached irrevocably to my grief. It wasn't a happy name anymore, as I had planned it to be, and it belonged to the child I had held—it was hers, officially or not.

To have saved her name for another child would have done that child an injustice as well. It was important that our next child be wanted for his or her own sake, not as a replacement. This was something the social worker impressed upon me and Dean. "When you have another child," she told us, "it won't be good to confuse that child with the one you lost. Do your mourning now; do it fully. For each couple, each person, that means something different. Ask yourselves what you need to do so you can be ready to welcome a new child."

Once we began to speak of the baby we had held as Amelia, Dean and I found she was less a chimera and more a daughter who had died. I didn't look away from her memory as much anymore; I looked directly at it and admitted that, after all, I would never have a living daughter named Amelia.

My greatest solace at this time was the prospect of another pregnancy, and I was eager to prove Dr. Kagan's optimism justified. Recommending that I get pregnant soon, within two months of the operation if possible, Dr. Barrie's instructions meshed with my impatience; she thought it likely that I would develop more fibroids, and she wanted me to get ahead of them, not give them a chance to grow. This winter, I kept telling myself, this winter will be a good time. Though I was scared of being pregnant so soon after surgery, the scar across my belly still raw, and the other incision still smarting, the one inside, the one a baby would push against and test, my sense of urgency ruled me.

But in Dean's case continuing grief produced hesitancy. He wasn't even certain he would ever want to try again. "You've got to let me consider both possibilities," he told me. "Don't make me feel I can't choose not to risk another loss."

When I pleaded, he demanded patience. "Don't push me. Give me time."

I lay beside him at night telling myself he had a right to refuse to try again, a right to be that afraid. But, just as it had before we were married, the thought that Dean and I might never have a child floated me into a black, empty space, like the thought of my own death. And now it was worse, even. Because now there had been Amelia, and if I never had another child, I would be mothering a ghost for the rest of my life.

2

I sat up, hanging my legs over the doctor's end of the examining table, letting the tension flow from my muscles. It was six weeks after my surgery, and Dr. Barrie had just announced that I was "doing beautifully," well enough to go back to work and to drive.

"You're really pleased?"

"Yes, very, you're healing just the way I like to see."

"What a relief. I never expect a good report from you." Dr. Barrie and I both laughed. "How's Dr. Kagan?"

"She's on leave now. She's due in a couple of weeks."

"I think I'll drop her a note. I'd like to thank her again."

"I'm sure she would appreciate that." Dr. Barrie stepped sideways towards the door. She paused there, and I got down from the table and reached for my underpants, draped over the chair by the sink. "I'm glad Dean drove you, because I did want to speak to the two of you. We got the autopsy report, and there's something in it I need to discuss with you."

I sat down in the chair. Autopsy report? They had done the autopsy months ago, early in the summer.

"I didn't even think that was an issue anymore. I thought there was nothing to find."

"Well, no, we didn't have a thorough report until now, and I do want to review it with you."

What on earth had they found? What's wrong, what's wrong, I wanted to ask, but didn't dare.

"I'll get dressed," I said. Whatever Dr. Barrie had to say, I didn't want to hear it alone. I wanted to be with Dean.

"The autopsy has given us an explanation of why your baby died." Dr. Barrie says this calmly, matter-of-factly, as though it's not a grenade thrown between me and Dean, about to explode. She tells us that our baby died either from Niemann-Pick disease or Gaucher's disease, both genetically inherited metabolic disorders. "Dr. Jakolski, a geneticist at the Mass. General lab, is still studying the fetal tissue to make the diagnosis definite, but he's fairly certain it was Gaucher's."

Dean and I exchange looks of disbelief; he takes my hand. "What is all this?" he asks. "You told us the baby's death was just bad luck, now you're telling us . . ."

"We did think it was just a random occurrence, but Dr. Jakolski's lab is quite sure now it was not. You must both be carriers for one of these diseases, which means that for any given pregnancy there is a 25 percent chance—one in four—of the baby having the disorder."

I begin to cry. (I don't want to cry, I'm sick of myself crying so much, but I can't help it, I give in, I'm rocking forward and back on the edge of my chair.) "Maybe they're wrong. How do they know for sure?"

"Marion, Dr. Jakolski's lab has been examining the tissue they took from your baby, examining it with very sophisticated techniques, using electron microscopy, and it has the characteristics associated with these disorders. These are enzyme disorders, like Tay-Sachs, which means that a specific enzyme necessary for breaking down food is missing. You must understand, Dr. Jakolski is not in doubt about whether it's one of these diseases; his only question at this point is which one, and when he knows, I'll ask you both to have your blood tested to confirm the finding. Carriers are easily identified, because their blood shows a lower than normal level of the enzyme. Your baby had none of the enzyme, which made it impossible for her to survive. Carriers like you have enough of the enzyme to lead normal lives, but a total lack . . . well, that's fatal."

Dr. Barrie draws a box on a piece of paper and divides it into four sections, drawing X's and O's to show the possible genetic combinations. "Do you remember your high school biology? Mendel's peas? You and Dean are XO, the O being the recessive gene. You're unharmed, but your enzyme level is not the normal XX level. For each pregnancy, there's a two in four chance of your baby being XO—a carrier like you; there's a one in four chance of your baby being XX—perfectly normal and not a carrier; but there's a one in four chance of OO. That's what your baby was."

"We sure have the luck, don't we?" I mumble.

"Why didn't Dr. Mertz ever mention Gaucher's?" Dean asks.

"I've spoken to Dr. Mertz, and he's as shocked by this diagnosis as I am. Gaucher's doesn't usually show up in utero, and he never even considered it."

Dr. Barrie explains that Gaucher's babies usually die in the first year or so of life. "Your child was really spared great agony. It was much better that she died as she did. Gaucher's babies can't digest properly. The brain is affected. The liver, the spleen. They're in constant pain and they can't see or hear you. They're vegetables."

"Why didn't the amniocentesis show anything?" Dean's voice is calm like Dr. Barrie's, but I can feel him flailing just under the surface. He asks the question I've been afraid to ask: "Can't they test for this?"

"They can, but they don't do it as a matter of routine. It has to be requested, and of course we didn't know we had any reason to make such a request in your case."

Some concealed corner of me is rejoicing, calculating,

saving a little space for hope—thinking, we haven't quite been blown to bits. But that's not the part that speaks, the part looking at Dr. Barrie. "So if I get pregnant and I'm tested, there's a one in four chance of needing an abortion at around twenty weeks. Going through another horror show. Like we've just been through." Dr. Barrie looks at me and nods.

"How definite is all this?" Dean asks. "Do we have any hope that it's not one of these genetic diseases?"

"No, don't expect that. It's almost certainly Gaucher's, though there's still a slight chance it's Niemann-Pick disease, but it is one or the other. Look, the good in all this is that we know now what happened, and it can be tested for."

"I don't feel good about any of it," I say. "Don't you think we should give up? Isn't that really what you're trying to let us know?"

"No, not at all. You've got an obstacle, but it's not insurmountable. If I thought you should give up, I'd tell you."

"Have you ever told a patient that?"

"Yes, I have. But I'm not ready to tell you that. Right now, Dr. Jakolski wants another fetal tissue sample, and I understand that Brigham and Women's has been slow to get him the tissue."

"They still have the baby's tissue?"

"Yes, some of the lung tissue was frozen and stored. I'm trying to hurry Brigham and Women's now, especially since you want to get pregnant fairly soon because of the fibroid situation. As soon as Dr. Jakolski has the tissue and determines which disease we're dealing with, you can go for your blood tests. Then I'll arrange for you to see him to discuss the implications of your being carriers. He'll tell you which family members should be tested in case they're planning to have children, and he can answer some of your questions better than I can. These diseases are very rare; we've never seen a case of either one of them here."

On leaving Dr. Barrie's office, Dean and I sit down in the lounge and hug each other. "How can this be happening to us?"

"I don't know," Dean says, "I don't know. The game has certainly changed."

And it had changed; it was no longer just a matter of getting pregnant again and hoping for the best. Now we would be knowingly taking a one in four gamble against our own genetic stuff. One in four. We knew what the "one" was like; we had just lived through it.

Apart, we wouldn't have had to play the game, but together, so long as we wanted a child born of the two of us, our flesh and blood, this was the only game we could play. For the first time, I wondered if it made sense to try again.

In the next few weeks, Dr. Jakolski determined that our baby had unquestionably died of Gaucher's, and blood tests confirmed that Dean and I are indeed carriers for that disease. How strange it was to learn this about ourselves; to learn how singularly each of us had been cursed and blessed at our conception, dealt this "bad gene," yet, by its pairing with a healthy gene, enabled to live. Had we never met, never fallen in love, never had our child, this mysterious fact of our biologies might have lurked unknown all our lives. No one in either of our families had ever heard the word "Gaucher's."

Giving me the results of the blood tests over the telephone, Dr. Barrie had other news, about a new type of genetic test, an experimental procedure—chorionic villus biopsy, it was called—being developed as an alternative to amniocentesis. "It's done much earlier than amniocentesis, at nine weeks," she explained, "and there's a project at Yale making it available to couples like you. I went to a conference last week where some of the Yale doctors spoke about this. If you want, I can get in touch with them for you."

"Will that test work for this disease?"

"That's what we need to find out. I'm not sure, but since they can test for Gaucher's through amniocentesis, my guess is that the villus biopsy can be used as well. I think you can let yourself be optimistic about it, if it makes you feel better, but don't count on it yet. Would you like me to contact them for you?"

"Yes, definitely."

In a few days, Dr. Barrie had the answer: the Yale program would be pleased to accept me and Dean, and Dr. Jakolski saw no reason why the villus sample couldn't be used to test for Gaucher's.

In spite of the fact that the procedure was still considered experimental and carried a higher risk of miscarriage than amniocentesis, Dr. Barrie thought it would make sense, under the circumstances, for us to use this new form of testing. "I think this method is really the method of the future," she told me. "Someday, I think, it will be generally available and even preferred to amniocentesis."

It was December by the time Dean and I met with Dr. Jakolski. He called us one day to ask if we would be willing to provide additional blood samples right away; there were important analyses he wanted to do before attending a meeting with other Gaucher's experts in Washington, D.C., the following week. Nothing that would affect us personally, he admitted, but important for the understanding of the disease. He was so eager to have the blood samples that he offered to come to our house for them. "I can spend a little time," he said, "and try to answer your questions." He was apologetic, careful not to be too insistent.

At seven-thirty the morning after his call Dean and I stood at our storm door watching him walk up the path from the driveway to the front steps. "My God, the mad scientist," I said.

Dr. Jakolski stepped carefully on the snowy flagstones, holding out in front of him, like some precious object of religious ritual, a tray of empty test tubes. He was so thin as to look gaunt, and his bushy eyebrows seemed to have just stuck to him, like pieces of wind-torn nest fallen from the bare maple over the walk. The shape of his face—so narrow it seemed you could fold it flat along the prominent ridge of his nose—reminded me of his hat, one of those boat-shaped Russian hats of black fur. His topcoat was open, and he had on a suit and tie; except for his plain white shirt, everything he wore was black.

At our kitchen table he set his tray down and draped his topcoat over a chair. His suit was baggy on his bony frame, and exhausted-looking, as though he asked too much of it, forced it to be a witness to too many strange occasions. "I was looking forward to meeting you all summer," he said, a remark which Dean and I mused over later as possibly indicating that Dr. Barrie had known about the Gaucher's problem much earlier but had decided to spare us the news until after my surgery.

While he washed his hands and got a needle ready, Dr. Jakolski answered some of our questions about Gaucher's. He recommended that our siblings be tested if they had any plans to have children. "Though it's highly unlikely, you understand, that their spouses will be carriers. Infantile Gaucher's, the type of Gaucher's your baby had, is the most severe form of the disease, and the most rare. There are other types as well; the most common generally goes unnoticed until middle age, when spleen problems develop. The infantile type is always fatal, within a year or so of birth. It rarely produces death in utero. There are only two other cases like yours in the world, that we know of."

Dr. Jakolski wrapped a piece of rubber tubing around my upper arm and felt for a vein by the crook of my elbow. "I haven't done this in a while," he said; but the needle was already in, and he was filling first one, then a second, then a third tube with blood.

"How many do you need?"

"Eight."

I grimaced and looked away. Looked up at Dean. He was leaning one hand on the kitchen counter, while with the other he drew out one end of his reddish mustache repeatedly between thumb and forefinger, a habit of his that seemed to be simultaneously a tranquilizer and an aid to thought. He was dressed for work, and he had taken off his suit jacket and rolled up one of his sleeves. Dr. Jakolski put a Band-Aid on my arm and I got up to give Dean my chair at the table. "Next victim."

While Dr. Jakolski prepared another needle, then jabbed it into Dean's arm and began filling eight more tubes with blood, he went on talking, with a zealot's enthusiasm for his subject. "Gaucher's is more common in Jews. Like Tay-Sachs. About one in thirty Ashkenazi Jews—East European Jews—carries the Tay-Sachs gene; the incidence of Gaucher's may actually be somewhat higher than that."

"Dean, maybe you're really Jewish."

"No kidding, maybe it's the German blood, back there on my father's mother's side."

Dr. Jakolski laughed. "Actually, from past experience we would not expect a Jew to be a carrier for the infantile form of the disease. That adds to the oddity of your case."

"What's the chance of a non-Jew being a carrier for Gaucher's?" Dean asked.

"Again, the incidence is similar as for Tay-Sachs, but perhaps a bit more frequent. For Tay-Sachs, it's one in three hundred; Gaucher's may be more like one in two hundred."

"Better give me an extra Band-Aid," Dean said, starting to roll up his sleeve.

Dr. Jakolski tidied the tray of test tubes and supplies and washed his hands again. I poured glasses of juice and bowls of cereal for me and Dean ("No thanks, nothing for me," Dr. Jakolski insisted) and felt myself hesitating to put them on the table, so close to the drawn blood.

"Go ahead," Dean said, laughing at me. "Just don't knock that blood over. My arm's sore."

"Dr. Barrie tells me you're considering the villus biopsy," said Dr. Jakolski.

"Amniocentesis comes too late," I responded, as if needing to explain. "I was that far along last time when the baby came, so I know what . . ."

"I agree with you. And with Dr. Barrie. It's your best way to go."

"I was reading an article about it. By a pediatrician. She said it may cause birth defects and prematurity. She says to stick with amnio."

"She's thinking about babies, not their mothers."

"That was my response," said Dean.

"Anyway," Dr. Jakolski continued, "I don't know that there's any evidence of such problems. The thing to do is to speak to them at Yale yourself. Find out."

At the front door, Dr. Jakolski thanked us. "Call me any time with questions. Don't hesitate. I want to help in any way I can. Nothing would make me happier than to see you two with a healthy baby."

I opened the storm door to let him through with the tray of blood-filled tubes. "One thing for sure," he said, "you don't want to have a child with Gaucher's." He paused. "There's a couple in Vermont right now. Their baby is almost a year old. I visited them a few weeks ago." He shook his head slowly. "It's a dreadful disease." Under the disheveled brows, his eyes focused inward for a moment on that other home: the parents, the dying infant. "Compared to them, you're lucky."

CHAPTER 6

TRYING AGAIN

1

In 1984, only three medical centers in the United States had approval from the National Institutes of Health to perform villus biopsies on women hoping to carry their pregnancies to term; it was a stroke of luck for me and Dean that Yale's School of Medicine, a relatively short drive from Boston, was one of them. Most medical centers, including Mass. General in Boston, were as yet permitted only to "practice" the biopsy technique on women planning abortions.

When I called Dr. Embry, the gynecologist performing the biopsies at Yale, I had to tell myself to be realistic, not to expect the world. The call went well. Dr. Embry gave me as much reassurance as I had dared to hope for. There were, she said, no known risks of prematurity or birth defects associated with the villus biopsy, no evidence whatsoever that these were problems. The technique used at Yale, the so-called Italian technique, had been used internationally on over a hundred biopsies and was the safest method, with the simplest equipment and the lowest risk of infection. This point about infection was important, Dr. Embry said, because a uterine infection would mean a lost pregnancy and possibly a hysterectomy. But she didn't think I should worry much about this. Infections had occurred only in a few hospitals abroad, and never at Yale, and were more likely caused by something in the hospital environment than by the procedure.

Of the thirty or so biopsies performed by Dr. Embry, two had involved women not planning abortions, both of whom were so far progressing normally in their pregnancies. "The real risk you need to consider isn't prematurity or birth defects," Dr. Embry told me, "it's miscarriage." That didn't scare me much. Dean and I had already decided that of the risks confronting us miscarriage was the lesser one, the more acceptable.

I had my questions in front of me, written out on a pad. There were so many. "What I don't understand is why the procedure isn't *always* harmful. I mean, you're taking part of the placenta."

"For one thing, we're taking a very minute portion of the placenta, about 1/500th of the existing tissue. Also, we think the body may replace the villi, the little hairlike projections we remove." Dr. Embry's voice was thin and squiggly, friendly, not looping around the question, not trying to make it my last one. I was scribbling furiously, taking notes to share later with Dean.

I was worried about the procedure for getting into the program, but Dr. Embry put my mind at ease on this point too. If I became pregnant, acceptance would be automatic, my genetic problem and my history of second trimester loss each being sufficient grounds for acceptance. I needed only to call Dr. Embry once I knew I was pregnant.

"We'll perform the biopsy early in the morning." Dr. Embry spoke as though my getting pregnant was a safe assumption. "You'll probably want to arrive in New Haven the day before. We can help you with hotel arrangements when the time comes. Once the biopsy is completed, we require only that you rest here long enough for us to do an ultrasound one hour after the procedure. You'll also need to have an ultrasound done after six hours, but your radiologist in Cambridge can do that. As far as the tissue sample is concerned, the chromosome testing, the standard test usually done through amniocentesis, will be handled here at Yale. For the Gaucher's test, we'll use Dr. Jakolski's lab. We can send him the sample by courier or let you carry it back."

"Won't I be in pain after the biopsy? Or too tired to travel?"

"Not especially. Most women are ready to get up and walk around that first hour, before we've even done the ultrasound. You can expect some spotting afterwards, but that's a natural result of tampering with the cervix or placenta during pregnancy. There is, as I said, a risk of miscarriage, so you would need to let your doctor know right away if you had any excessive bleeding."

(How would I know if the bleeding was excessive? Would I? What if I panicked?) "Do I have to come for a preliminary visit?"

"No, you'll need a preliminary ultrasound and a routine gonorrhea test, nothing more. You can take care of all that up there and have your doctor phone me the results."

As for the crucial question of whether the villus tissue could be used to test for Gaucher's, Dr. Embry said that Dr. Jakolski was the one to ask. "He's the expert. I have a positive answer from his assistant, but I'd like the question put to him directly."

"Dr. Barrie did ask him. So did we. He says he can do it."

"Good. Then assume we can."

No doctor anywhere in the world had ever used the villus biopsy to test for Gaucher's.

Dean and I agreed that if I became pregnant again we would go to Yale for a biopsy. Since it was in that context that we considered a second pregnancy, it's impossible to be sure what we would have done if we had had to rely on amniocentesis. I recall us saying more than once that without the biopsy a second pregnancy would have been out of the question; but I wonder whether we wouldn't have mustered our courage all the same.

As it was, even with the biopsy available, Dean couldn't decide at first whether he wanted to try again. I knew I did.

"Take the time you need," Dr. Barrie told us, inexplicably abandoning her opposition to a prolonged hiatus. "Even if you wait until next fall you'll be okay." Dean and I greeted this change of instructions with relief. (We suspected our social worker of having been at work behind the scenes, though Dr. Barrie denied it.) For my part, I was pleased to hear that a few months' wait would not so dramatically increase my risk of developing new fibroids as Dr. Barrie had at first suggested; and I was hopeful that Dean, less pressured now, would begin to feel a little lighter, more expansive, more ready.

As January, the anniversary of Amelia's conception, slipped by, I convinced myself superstitiously that it would have been a bad month to begin trying again anyway. But "next fall" was a longer reprieve than I would have wished for, depressingly far off. Time was passing and I was no closer to being a mother. A year before, I had been thinking, thirty-five, at least when the baby comes I won't be any older than that; now I had only a few months until April and my thirty-sixth birthday. And in May it would be a full year since the delivery.

I didn't need to tell Dean that I was counting on him to come around. He knew. He knew I refused to believe we would never try again.

And then, in February, he was suddenly willing. He rejoined me, as it were, after several months of partial retreat.

Fearing that it might take many more months for me to conceive, I began charting my temperature again, knowing that the longer it took the more convinced I would become that my surgery had created some obstacle to conception. Gradually I seized upon a secret deadline, a date with magic in it. I wanted to be pregnant if not by my birthday then by Memorial Day, the anniversary of Amelia's death.

As much as if she had lived, I told time—tolled time, you might say—by Amelia's milestones, the date of her conception, the date of her death, the date she had been "due." I marked her history, the ephemeral promise of it and the crushing disappointment of it, with a series of bitter memorials. These were not dates remembered by family and friends. Their significance was strictly private.

When my mother called me the day after Memorial Day, I doubt that she was thinking at all of the special meaning that weekend held for me and Dean. She would have been surprised, shocked, to know that we had consciously prepared for that weekend, me by finishing the letter I had been writing to Amelia, Dean by promising to read it. Indeed, like the rest of our relatives, my mother didn't even know we had named our child.

She was calling with other matters on her mind. Uppermost was the news that my mother-in-law from my first marriage had died.

I had last seen my ex-mother-in-law the year before on my trip to Florida, when I had known that she was ill and that I might not see her again. It was then that she had surprised me with the blanket she had crocheted for my baby. "You look wonderful," she had declared. "Pregnancy agrees with you." Later, when I called to tell her about the stillbirth, knowing she too had once lost a baby girl, I wanted to reassure her about the blanket. "Don't worry," I said, "I'm still going to use it someday."

"I have that baby blanket she made," I said to my mother now, bursting into tears. And then, careful not to mention the letter or to reveal that the baby had a name, I reminded my mother that Dean and I had just passed the anniversary of our baby's death.

"Maybe you should think about adopting," she proposed. "I have a friend whose daughter just adopted, and she's in seventh heaven."

My mother's offering this advice didn't surprise me; the response was common among relatives and friends who wanted to help. So simple, so wonderful, the suggestion implied, just the solution. But the very word made me nervous, defensive. Dean and I didn't want to adopt; we wanted to "have our own"—and we still could. In fact, my period was a few days late, and I was thinking that perhaps Dean and I had met my magic deadline after all.

"I'm hoping I may be pregnant," I told my mother. I hadn't wanted to mention this to her, but here I was, pitting my slim hope against the idea of adopting.

"That's wonderful, dear," my mother said, "I'll keep my fingers crossed. Can I tell you about Nery?"

Nery? What, I wondered, could my mother have in mind to tell me about my sister-in-law? She was five months pregnant with her second child, and I had told my mother from the beginning of her pregnancy that I couldn't bear to hear much about it. Something must be wrong, I thought. "Nery? What do you mean," I asked, "is something wrong?"

"No, nothing's wrong. She got good news today. The amniocentesis report came back."

I don't want to hear, I thought, I don't want to hear.

"Everything's perfect."

I tried desperately to find the correct emotion, the gladness I was supposed to feel for my sister-in-law and my brother; but it wasn't there anymore.

"It's a healthy little girl," my mother was saying.

A girl! Ever since hearing Nery was pregnant, just let it be a boy, I had thought, please, God, let it be a boy for them, not a girl. Incredibly, the baby was due October 7, the same date Amelia had been given.

"They're very excited."

"Yes, I'm sure they are."

Unfortunately for me, my mother fell into that category of relatives and friends who proved insensitive—sometimes joltingly so—to what Dean and I were going through. Her insensitivity was partly the result of ignorance about pregnancy loss (as she herself, passionately apologetic, has since explained to me), but it was also a defense against her own disappointment. Such glimmerings as she may have had of how deeply I was grieving she did not want to fully see or understand, because my child's dying had pained her too. Further complicating our relationship was a subtle undercurrent of blaming that passed in both directions, each of us irrationally holding the other responsible for the lost child and grandchild. I was even perversely jealous of my mother's relationship with me—why should *she* have had a fine, healthy daughter, and not I? Insensitive as she was, I thought, she didn't deserve a daughter; *I* would never have been so hurtful to *mine*.

What I needed was to be indulged for a while, to have allowances made for me. This, I now believe, is the prerogative of the victim of any tragedy, and only the victim can define the need—the kind of allowances that must be made, the length of time the indulgence is required. If I couldn't bear to hear the details of my sister-in-law's pregnancy; if I couldn't remain long in a room where my mother and a family friend swapped stories about their grandchildren; if I couldn't bring myself to shop for a birthday gift for my six year old nephew; if these alterations in behavior were my automatic protection against insupportable depression, no excuses were required. My mother tried to appreciate this, she tried to indulge me, and sometimes she succeeded, but this was not something she managed easily; periodically, her efforts collapsed in ill-timed comments and demanding, faultfinding phone calls, and I retreated from her more and more.

The growing distance between us came, ironically, at the time in my life when I most needed to feel a family closeness. Having failed to extend my life into a new generation of family, I needed more than ever the family I already had.

The discovery of the genetic disorder reinforced, for Dean as well as for me, the two conflicting emotions: the longing for family closeness, and the simultaneous sense of isolation. Both Dean's mother and mine reacted to the genetic revelation as though it was an accusation; his mother seemed defensive, and unsympathetic to our depression; my mother was preoccupied with the origin of the "bad" gene, hastening to observe that it must have come from my father's side of the family. In a sense, Dean and I had become family freaks. There was a differentness about us, a taint, that made everyone else nervous.

Because my brother and his wife, Nery, had wanted to have a second child, and were just feeling ready at about the time Dean and I learned of the Gaucher's problem, I had written them a long letter explaining as much as I understood, and passing along Dr. Jakolski's recommendation that my brother have his blood tested. I hated writing that letter. I'm not especially close to my brother and his wife, and I felt as though forced against my instincts to show them something painful and private; I felt the way a witness must feel lifting a skirt or opening a blouse in a courtroom to show a smear of purple bruises. I knew that my brother and his wife would come out all right; they already had one child, and they would succeed in having another. I never doubted this, and I was jealous. It isn't that I wished them to have my problem. It's just that I didn't wish me to have the problem either. I resented the relief they must inevitably feel when they learned they hadn't been marked like me and Dean. How could they not be relieved to be different from us? And different they were. My brother's blood test showed him to be a Gaucher's carrier, but his wife, as statistically one would expect, was normal; their worries were over. By January, Nery had conceived, and when, because of her age, she had gone for a routine amniocentesis, Gaucher's hadn't even been an issue.

For Dean, the isolation from family was deepened by his parents' adherence to Catholic doctrine on abortion. His mother had said on more than one occasion, "Abortion is murder." Dean told his parents nothing of our plans to go to Yale for the biopsy in the event of a second pregnancy; nothing of our intentions to abort a fetus known to have Gaucher's; and nothing of how close we had come to proceeding with an abortion during my hospitalization with Amelia. Dean's parents weren't even aware of my ever having had amniocentesis, though I believe they may have suspected more than they let on. They didn't ask questions that might produce the wrong answers. Though they plainly wished for me to have a second pregnancy, they never asked— and in this they were strikingly different from other close relatives and friends—whether there was any form of genetic testing for Gaucher's. Their omission made me angry; I never had the feeling they were willing to acknowledge, truly acknowledge, our predicament. Their religious rules were so important to them that their compassion and understanding sometimes seemed confined to a box of a certain shape; the rules came first, before the urge to shield, to protect, their son.

Like the mortal in the fairy tale who makes a wish but fails to accurately specify the terms, I was indeed pregnant on Memorial Day, as the first year of mourning ended and the second year began. A blood test on June 7 confirmed this. But from the beginning there were problems.

The results of my blood test were not what they should have been. I was pregnant, but my "beta-sub" count—a measure of the level of the so-called beta subunit of a particular hormone that increases during pregnancy—was seven hundred when it should have been in the thousands. Dr. Barrie was afraid I might be having an ectopic pregnancy, possibly due to scarring from my surgery. I was in danger not only of losing the pregnancy but of requiring another operation.

The results of a second test a few days later were "encouraging," according to Dr. Barrie, but still not what they ought to have been. She now thought the pregnancy probably wasn't ectopic, but she wanted me to see Dr. Abram for an ultrasound exam in order to be sure. "If this is ectopic," she warned me, "I'll have to put you right into the hospital."

At the exam, Dean and I couldn't tell what Dr. Abram was looking at among the streaks on the screen, but she said she could see a fetus and a heartbeat; my pregnancy was not ectopic. She saw no fibroids either. What did concern her, however, though only a little, was the peripheral location of the fetus, the way in which the placenta was crowded, as I understand it, into a corner of the uterus, rather than being attached nearer the center. "This may not be a problem at all. It's nothing you should worry yourself about. But we'll want to keep an eye on it."

During the week following the exam, a third blood test produced a perfectly normal result, bolstering my confidence and restoring to its place of primary concern the question to be answered at Yale. But then on June 20 I was shaken again. I was driving along Mt. Auburn Street in Cambridge, when, suddenly aware of a warm liquid pooling between my legs, I discovered that I was sitting in a puddle of blood. I drove myself to the emergency unit at Mt. Auburn Hospital, fortuitously only a few hundred yards away. I didn't miscarry that day, as I at first believed I would, but the episode went unexplained, and I, along with Dean, who rushed from his office to the hospital, was unnerved by it as I tried to ready myself for the trip to Yale.

The appointment at Yale was set for Monday, July 2, when I would be almost ten weeks pregnant. In the mail I had received a consent form I was supposed to review and bring along with me.

CHORIONIC VILLOUS BIOPSY FOR ANTENATAL DIAGNOSIS, it said. CONSENT FOR PARTICIPATION IN A RESEARCH PROJECT, YALE UNIVERSITY SCHOOL OF MEDICINE—YALE-NEW HAVEN HOSPITAL. Just the heading made me nervous. Yet I was relieved to have the form in my hands and to know Yale wasn't backing out; I had, after all, hazarded this pregnancy on the strength of Dr. Embry's promise.

I read the two pages in dread of what they might say, not wanting to waver in my decision:

> You are invited to participate in a research effort to study the process of chorionic villous biopsy as a method of prenatal diagnosis of genetic disease in a developing fetus, and to study the risks of this new procedure and how accurate it is as a diagnostic method. Chorionic villous biopsy means the withdrawing of a tiny sample of the developing placenta (afterbirth) from within your womb when you are 7 to 13 weeks pregnant (dating from last normal menstrual period). . . .
>
> The biopsy will be done with you lying on an obstetric examining table with your legs supported by stirrups. After thorough cleansing of your vagina, a thin tube (catheter) with a syringe attached will be advanced through the cervix (neck of the womb) to the placenta and a few villi will be removed. The biopsy procedure has only minimal discomfort associated with it and takes only a few minutes. After the biopsy you will have to stay for

3-4 hours for observation. We will be observing the biopsy with ultrasound while it is being done and we will
examine your pregnancy again with ultrasound before
you leave the hospital. . . .

Chorionic villous biopsy is new and risks are not well
established as yet. There is a small risk (less than 5
percent) of infection within your womb. We will be taking precautions against this but if it should occur, it
would require ending the pregnancy and treating you in
the hospital with antibiotics. There is a remote chance
that infection or bleeding could lead to decreased subsequent fertility or could necessitate removal of your womb.

Risks to the developing baby are largely unknown at
this time. Experience in Europe and Asia with chorionic
villous biopsy is limited to less than 300 pregnancies and
only a few babies have yet been born. These babies have
been normal and the babies that are still in the womb
appear to be developing normally. Miscarriage has complicated about 1 in 10 of these pregnancies, however.
Some of these miscarriages would have occurred anyway
(lots of miscarriages occur in the first trimester of pregnancy), but some were caused by the biopsy procedure.
How large this risk is for you cannot yet be stated with
any accuracy. We believe it will be less than 1 in 10 based
on our own work and work from other medical centers.

Dean and I told almost no one about my pregnancy—
fewer than ten close friends, and no relatives. It was
impossible for us to feel the same anticipatory joy we
had felt during my first pregnancy, and there were few
people we trusted to understand why we were holding
in our hope so tight, like an unreleased gulp of air. We
wanted to wait before we shared our news, to wait
until we could do so with the benefit of a good report
from Yale. That would be the time to bring our families
and the rest of our friends into the circle of our happi-
ness. It was the tidiest approach, and it assumed that
we would receive a good report. We never considered
the extreme isolation we would have to bear if things
went poorly.

*   *   *

Four days before I was scheduled to go to Yale, Dr. Abram examined me again. She was able to see the fetus, as before, and this time even I could detect the pulse. "Do you see the heartbeat, Dean?" I asked.

Yes, he saw it too.

We reminded Dr. Abram that we would be back again Monday afternoon for a follow-up sonogram upon our return from Yale. I couldn't tell what she thought of our plan to participate in the Yale program, but I guessed that she liked being connected with the experiment. "Will you be seeing Dr. Paulson?" she asked. "We went to medical school together."

Dr. Abram rarely said anything that wasn't a direct comment about the image on the screen, so her inquiry surprised and pleased me, and I was sorry to be unable to oblige her. "No, there's no Dr. Paulson in this project, just Dr. Embry, who will be doing the biopsy, and Dr. Cooper, the director."

"Well, if you meet Dr. Paulson there, say hello for me. And good luck."

I remember us driving into New Haven early Sunday evening, Dean at the wheel, me trying to direct him, calling off the names of cross streets. Part of me had a tourist's curiosity and enthusiasm. I wanted to find the hotel, take a walk, choose a place to have dinner. But it was impossible to forget for a moment the purpose of our trip, impossible to relax and stop thinking about Monday morning, impossible not to wonder whether the detailed arrangements we had worked out with Yale over the past few weeks would proceed smoothly.

Because this was going to be the first time the villus biopsy had ever been used to test for Gaucher's, there was no proven path to follow, and Dr. Barrie and Dr. Cooper hadn't automatically agreed on the best way to proceed. Who should test the placental tissue had become a matter of controversy. At my first acceptance into the project, the assumption by both sides had been that Dr. Jakolski would do the testing. The staff at Yale had readied his lab by providing a control sample, tissue from a healthy placenta that had been aborted, so Dr. Jakolski could establish, in advance of my test, enzyme levels for a normal biopsy. But the week before my trip to Yale, Dr. Cooper expressed a preference for sending the villus sample to a lab at Mt. Sinai Hospital in New York, a lab Dr. Cooper had used for previous biopsies. Dr. Barrie maintained that the tissue ought to be tested by Dr. Jakolski, because it was he who had discovered the cause of Amelia's death and whose lab had tested my blood and Dean's, and it was he who was most accessible to us. Dr. Barrie and he already knew each other, and Dean and I could deliver the biopsy material to him ourselves, rather than entrusting it to a courier.

It had been decided, after numerous phone calls, including a conference call Dean and I had made to Dr. Cooper, that the test for Gaucher's would be conducted by Dr. Jakolski, and a backup test would be conducted at Mt. Sinai if, as was likely, the villus sample was adequate to allow testing by a second lab.

Now I worried: what if the labs got inconsistent results? Was that possible?

Checking into the Colony Inn, a hotel that gave us a discounted rate as outpatients at Yale-New Haven Hospital, I felt as though I had been handed someone else's script. No matter how many times you read in the newspapers about someone traveling to a strange city for some new medical treatment, you never expect to make that kind of pilgrimage yourself. But here we were.

It was a warm, sunny morning when Dean and I walked from the hotel to the hospital. The storefronts and apartment buildings were depressing and uninteresting, the way I remembered New Haven from an earlier visit. Eight years had gone by since then, eight years! I had still been married to my first husband, hadn't even met Dean, hadn't any idea how elusive motherhood would be when I finally really wanted it.

.At least the procedure would soon be over. My mind was racing ahead to the drive back, the trip to Mass. General's genetics lab, where Dr. Jakolski's assistant would be expecting us, the visit to Dr. Abram at four-thirty. It seemed such a long path before I could lie down at home and comfort myself with having survived the day without losing my pregnancy. Then, within a week, we would have an answer.

I always tensed before doctors' appointments, but this was worse than usual. The word "experimental" kept flashing in my mind like a warning on a highway. It seemed incredible that we were there, that we were going through with this, that we had no acceptable choice; and that my pregnancy had become an event of significance in medical circles. (In spite of ourselves, Dean and I took a certain pride in my being a medical "first"; we had been shy about confessing this to each other, it seemed such a perverse expression of our egos.)

I liked Dr. Embry the minute she introduced herself. She was too skinny to look important, and her high forehead and narrow nose were softened by the kindness, the searching intelligence, of her blue eyes. As she ushered me and Dean into her office, speaking to us in a serious, breathy voice, it was evident that her patients' troubles kept her in a constant state of nervous concern and excitement. Her brown hair, hanging in limp waves to her shoulders, seemed to have collapsed from an excess of commotion, like a fallen cake.

Seated behind the large wooden desk that almost filled her small office, Dr. Embry looked like a shrinking Alice. She handed me a copy of the project's consent form to sign; and because I would need a full bladder for the ultrasound, she asked me to drink as many cups as possible from a quart carton of cold orange juice standing on her desk. While I drank the juice, she gave me and Dean a chance to ask last minute questions about the biopsy and to reconfirm our plans for delivering the tissue sample to Dr. Jakolski.

After assuring me that Dean could be with me during the biopsy, Dr. Embry opened her office door and led the way down the hall, toward an open door on the other side. I felt the way I do sometimes in dreams: caught up in a flow of events that can't be stopped; frightened but curious.

Half of the room we entered was a wide, empty space with nothing but a clothes locker and supply shelves along the walls. The examining table and ultrasound equipment stood farther in, nearer the windows. Sunlight filtered through the gray curtains, making shadowy patterns in the curtain folds and casting a watery shine over the paper-covered surface of the table.

A man in a white jacket was fiddling with the equipment, making some adjustment to the controls. "This is Dr. Paulson," Dr. Embry announced. "He'll be interpreting the sonogram while I take the sample."

"'Oh, Dr. Paulson! Dr. Abram asked me to say hello to you."

He pressed his full lips together thoughtfully, at first seeming not to recognize the name. Then, in a distracted way, "Oh, of course. Sure. Tell her regards."

I stepped out of my underpants and lay down on the table, raising my skirt above my abdomen while Dr. Embry spread a sheet over my legs. Dean leaned against the wall, near the foot of the table, not near enough for me to reach him with my hand. Dr. Embry was standing close to the table, on the same side, and Dr. Paulson stood opposite, on my right, by the ultrasound screen. My bladder was just beginning to feel full as Dr. Embry rubbed my abdomen with gel and began to press against me with the sensor.

Time slowed almost to a halt as I waited for Dr. Paulson to find the image he needed and to instruct

Dr. Embry to proceed with the biopsy. I knew that at any moment Dr. Embry would tell me to let my knees fall open, and I wanted only for that moment to come quickly and for the invasion, as I kept imagining it, with its sharp, unpredictable pain, to be done with.

But the pressing and pressing on my abdomen, near and even on my incision, continued, and Dr. Embry didn't tell me to let my knees fall open.

It was Dr. Paulson who spoke to me first. "Do you see this round area?" he asked, pointing to a striated area the size of a quarter on the screen. "You've got a cyst on your ovary."

I couldn't believe what I was hearing. What's he talking about, I thought, groping for a reassuring theory. "Dr. Barrie said the corpus luteum is swollen. Is that what you mean?"

"No. It's a cyst, a good-sized one." Dr. Paulson reminded me of a television weatherman I once knew who loved pointing out funnel clouds on his satellite map, loved the image's potential to frighten.

I looked at Dean to see if he was scared too, and he was.

"Look," I told Dr. Paulson, with a pleading, not a commanding, tone, while his half-grin and the moist satisfaction in his eyes made me hate him, "I've been through a lot. I can't handle this. You're going to have to slow down." It's cancer, I was thinking. He's going to tell me I have cancer. My panic was itself like one of those twisters; I'm sure the doctors felt it spinning between them. Neither of them spoke or moved.

"I just had fibroid surgery last September, and now you're telling me I've got a cyst?"

"It's not something to worry about," Dr. Paulson said finally. "Lots of women get these during pregnancy. It should go away afterwards."

Why the fuck didn't you say so in the first place, I thought. And my mind buzzed with questions. Why hadn't Dr. Barrie mentioned a cyst? What if, like my fibroid, it didn't go away? What harm might it cause during my pregnancy?

"How come Dr. Barrie and Dr. Abram never noticed any cyst?"

"I don't know, maybe it just wasn't there yet."

"But Marion saw Dr. Abram four days ago," Dean said.

"I don't know why she didn't see it. But it's there now."

I tried to calm myself, to ready myself for the biopsy, to put this business about the cyst out of my mind. It can wait, I told myself. You'll have plenty of time to worry about it later. He shouldn't have mentioned it now, there was no need.

"Signs of oligohydramnios."

"Yes, I can see that."

Dr. Embry and Dr. Paulson were talking across me. I was just beginning to wonder what their conversation meant, when Dr. Embry addressed me in a gentle, soothing voice that put me on a new level of alert. "I'm afraid we can't proceed, Marion." Dean stepped forward toward the table. I reached for his hand.

"What do you mean?" I asked. My eyes were staring in a panicky way I could feel; they were like two prickling cats, cornered, ready to spring. I was breathing fast. "Why not?"

"Marion, the placenta isn't the size it should be."

I turned toward the screen. The vague shapes, the speckly gray and white striations, told me nothing.

"Are you sure? How can you tell? Everything was fine when I saw Dr. Abram."

"We're sure. At nine and a half weeks, there should be more there. The fetus looks right for nine and a half weeks, but the placenta is definitely abnormal."

I began sobbing. Abnormal. Abnormal. We're in trouble again. "Can't you at least try?"

"We can't, Marion, we really can't. You would miscarry. There's hardly any placenta there."

Hardly any placenta there? How can it live? How can
it be nourished?

"How can it live, then?" I hear myself asking.

"Well, it can go on for a while, but if the condition
continues, the fetus will be harmed."

For me, the center never holds, never gets it right.
Why does my body betray me? Why?

"Will it die?"

"That depends on whether this problem turns around.
But I have to be honest with you, damage may already
have been done."

Dr. Embry is the one answering me. I want Dr.
Paulson to go away. I feel as though I'm a specimen to
him, a salamander on a rock. My grief, it seems, doesn't
touch him.

"Why don't you lie here awhile," Dr. Embry suggests. "Then you can come into my office and we'll talk
before you go. I'll speak to Dr. Cooper."

"I'll come in now. I don't want to lie here."

"Are you sure you're able to?"

"Yes, I'll be there in just a minute."

After Dr. Embry and Dr. Paulson go out, I stand up,
holding Dean's arm, and put on my underpants, and
smooth down my skirt. Dean and I hug each other,
and I keep thinking, how can we go home now, with
nothing accomplished and all unknown? Where are we
headed?

"You should wait till the end of the week, then have
another sonogram." Dr. Embry holds her chin in the
cup of her hand and looks at me and Dean pityingly.
"Maybe this problem will correct itself. This is an unusual condition. We don't see it very often, and it's
difficult to predict its course." She sits close to us, in
front of her desk, so close her knees almost touch
mine. I don't understand the long technical name she
gives to my condition, and neither Dean nor I bother to
ask. "We can perform the biopsy for up to twelve
weeks, so there's time, at least two weeks. Have Dr.

Abram talk to Dr. Paulson, and if they decide you're all right, we'll fit you in again. Please stay in touch with me. Let me know what's going on."

A red-winged blackbird rising swiftly at an angle out of tall grasses and scruffy trees. I always think of that blackbird—the flash of red on black scared out of the dense brush—when I think of that afternoon. Dean and I couldn't bear to go straight home when we left New Haven, and the one plan we could think of that seemed appropriate to the moment was for us to find a beach and take a walk by the ocean. From the Rhode Island map, we selected a beach neither of us had been to before, Misquamicut, and when we got there it turned out to be a perfect choice. We parked our car and walked on the grass along the side of the road to reach the entrance to the beach; and that was when we scared the blackbird out of the cricket-filled coolness of the brush. In the open it was hot and bright. And that bird flew up where I could see the red flash in the bright light and be reminded that what I loved about life was still there, outside my despair.

Walking along the water's edge, listening to the rush of the waves, surveying the clean stretch of sand that extended for miles, fairly deserted without the week-end crowds, Dean and I didn't talk much; we didn't have to. Our sadness passed between us, and into the sand and into the light, that dazzlingly white beach light. The scene was the only imaginable one open enough to receive our disappointment. I'm not a religious person in the traditional sense of the word, but I know there was a living love and sympathy there that we sought and that we needed, to get us through the rest of the day. I can't imagine how we could have gone home had we not first taken that walk along the beach.

When I called Dr. Barrie from home late that afternoon, she put my mind at ease about the cyst—it was, in spite of Dr. Paulson's leading me to believe otherwise, no more than the enlarged corpus luteum I already knew about, perfectly normal, certain to disappear when my pregnancy was over, if not before—but my prospects for the pregnancy, that was another matter.

"What's the word they used to describe my pregnancy?" I asked her. "Some long technical word."

"Oliogohydramnios?"

"That's it. What does it mean?"

"Oligo—little; too little. Hydro—water; fluid. It's a Greek word. Too little fluid. There's not enough fluid in the sac. This is a condition we rarely see. It's unusual for this to have happened. Very unusual."

"Is it linked to the bleeding I had?"

"I don't think so. Unless, perhaps, they're both linked to the peripheral location of the fetus."

"Why didn't Dr. Abram notice a problem? Don't you think I should go to someone else?"

"I don't know why she didn't see a problem. Perhaps it wasn't advanced enough then. Or perhaps she wasn't looking for the same thing as the people at Yale. You just won't find a more respected radiologist, though. It wouldn't make sense to send you to someone else."

"Do you think it will get better? The amount of fluid?"

"I don't think we can predict. You should wait until you see Dr. Abram."

"Dr. Embry says this can be linked to serious birth defects—kidney damage, heart damage, lung damage."

"Yes, it can."

"Why is this happening to us? After all we've been through?"

"I don't know. There's no connection. It's just terrible luck."

In the days that followed, Dean and I were worn down by the trap we were in as surely as if we had been two struggling animals in irons. Until I returned to Dr. Abram that Friday, even as Dean and I tried to prepare ourselves for the worst news, that nothing had changed, we tried to believe that there would be a change, a change so dramatic that the danger of fetal damage would be minimized and the biopsy and subsequent Gaucher's report would again become our one big concern. We speculated silently every moment of the day, and wearing as it had been from the first for us to know about my pregnancy and yet be unable to fully rejoice in it, now the inner tension was even worse because the evils threatening us had multiplied. Dean and I both found it impossible to properly concentrate at our jobs, and we were the more alone in our distress because we had taken almost no one into our confidence. When we spoke to our parents and other relatives by phone, we pretended to be happy and well, and for Dean, who had confided in fewer friends than I, the isolation was nearly absolute. We began to feel that in his case, if not also in mine, we had carried our secretiveness too far.

When Dr. Abram examined me and told us that nothing had changed, we realized what a thin hope we had been grasping since our trip to Yale. The trap was not opening.

"I'm sorry," Dr. Abram said. "It's still not what it ought to be. The fetus is growing, but the sac isn't."

"Why didn't you point out a problem before we went to Yale?" Dean asked.

"I did notice that the sac was a bit small then, but I didn't think it was anything to worry about. I didn't see any cause for concern."

"What about now? Do you agree that it's a problem?"

"I agree that it's abnormal. The sac isn't growing the way it should. It's definitely smaller than it ought to be."

"And the placenta?"

"That's small too."

"So the biopsy still can't be done, is that what you're saying?"

"I'm afraid so. If they couldn't do it on Monday, they wouldn't be able to do it now either."

"We would like you to call Dr. Paulson and discuss it with him." Dean made the request he and I had agreed on beforehand.

"I will, but I don't think you should get your hopes up. On the other hand, don't give up. You can come back next week and we'll have another look."

"What for? Do these pregnancies usually change? Is there reason to expect it to?"

"They usually don't change. No."

"And then what happens?"

"They miscarry, sooner or later."

"Do they always miscarry?"

"No. I have seen one case of oligohydramnios where the pregnancy resulted in birth—very prematurely. Twenty-four weeks."

"Twenty-four weeks!" Dean's voice was raised. "That's the *best* scenario? Is that supposed to be encouraging? Was the child healthy?"

"I don't know about that."

"Isn't it true," I asked, "that the earlier in the pregnancy this problem begins, the greater the likelihood of damage?"

"Yes, I'd say that's so. If it happens later in pregnancy, we can try to induce delivery before the fetus is harmed."

"That other woman you mentioned, when did her problem begin?"

"I don't recall if it was this early, if that's what you're getting at."

"I don't hear anything encouraging here at all," Dean said.

"And what about the Gaucher's?" I asked. "We've got that to think of, too."

"Yes, I know," Dr. Abram said, "but since you've

already had one loss, I hate to see you terminate this pregnancy."

"And since we've already had one loss," Dean said, "I hate to see us go on with it."

My phone conversation with Dr. Embry was no more heartening.

"Is there any reason to expect a change?" I asked.

"To be honest with you, I think a change is unlikely. But you may want to wait."

"But you can't even do the test after next week, isn't that right?"

"Well, basically, yes. I'd say you have a week and a half left at the most. Then there's amniocentesis, of course."

"But the whole reason we planned the biopsy was to avoid the chance of needing a second trimester abortion. Anyhow, how can they do amniocentesis when there's so little fluid?"

"They might not be able to."

"Why won't you do the biopsy? I've been so grateful to you people for letting me in the program, I hate to sound hostile now that things aren't working out, but aren't you people at Yale really just worried that I'll ruin your sample, screw up your results?"

Dr. Embry answered me gently, without anger. "Marion, no, that's really not it. We simply can't do the biopsy. There's so little tissue there, you'll miscarry. You'll definitely miscarry. It's not as though we have a choice."

"Oh . . . I see. I really hadn't understood that. Do you have any idea why this is happening to me?"

"No, not really, but I find myself wondering if perhaps this could be another Gaucher's baby. It's not impossible that the Gaucher's might cause this. I'm just theorizing."

"Dean and I are thinking of aborting the pregnancy. I know no one can make that decision for us, but will you tell me, does it seem reasonable to you, under the circumstances?"

"Yes, it seems reasonable. You're right, I can't tell you what to do, no one can, but if I were in your shoes, I'd certainly be thinking about an abortion."

That night I looked up "oligohydramnios" in the dictionary. "Deficiency of amniotic fluid," the dictionary said, "sometimes resulting in embryonic defect through adherence between embryo and amnion." That was a new one. The doctors hadn't even mentioned that the sac could stick to the fetus. It made sense, though.

"Quit looking at the dictionary," Dean told me. "That's not a medical text. Who knows how accurate it is?"

But what did it matter? There were enough statements from the doctors. "Heart damage." "Kidney damage." "We're not seeing enough motion." "Maybe due to lack of room in the sac." "Severe prematurity." "Permanent damage has very likely already occurred." "No, the condition isn't likely to change."

We had originally expected an answer about the Gaucher's problem by July 9, one week after the trip to Yale. But the day came with no answers, only questions. Dr. Barrie was talking in terms of our giving up on the biopsy and going on with the pregnancy in the hope of doing an amniocentesis at 16 weeks, if the low fluid level permitted a test. "We can still do an abortion then if we have to," she said. "Though the procedure is a higher-risk procedure than it would be now, it's still safe."

None of the doctors showed any signs of believing that we would still be able to have the biopsy at Yale. The sac was not developing normally and was not going to. That was the message.

On Tuesday, July 10, Dean and I went to see the social worker we had been seeing since Amelia's death.

It was impossible for me to talk to her without weeping. Dean's voice, on the other hand, had a determined calm about it, frozen, like the center of a lake that holds while jagged slabs of ice are breaking loose along the shore. "Dr. Barrie suggests we wait for another ultrasound," he explained, "but we feel it's like last time, when they knew things weren't going to change and they dragged out the torture with more examinations, more bad reports. The absolute best any doctor has suggested is that this baby, if it doesn't die first, will come prematurely, with a high likelihood of severe birth defects. And on top of that we can't test for Gaucher's at Yale and probably can't test later either. Anyhow, amniocentesis was never our plan; we were counting on an early answer from Yale. How can we continue with a pregnancy that's becoming a nightmare? How can we, especially after last time? Each day we wait it gets worse. Sometimes I feel like I'm losing my grip."

"The truth is," I said, thinking of how Dean had struggled within himself before agreeing to a second pregnancy, "if this pregnancy goes on any longer, we may never have the energy or the courage to try again. Our best hope for the future is to end this now."

Dr. Barrie agreed to perform the abortion herself instead of my going to a clinic. The first available date at Brigham and Women's Hospital was a week away, Thursday, July 19. So once again I found myself pregnant but facing an end instead of a beginning. Being in that condition while longing to have a child was almost unendurable; when I began running a fever, I wasn't surprised. I decided to stay home from work until my pregnancy was over, and I finally told my boss, the lawyer I did most of my work for, what I was going through. "Take all the time you need," she said.

That Tuesday, when my mother called to ask why she hadn't heard from me lately, I told her the reason.

"I'm pregnant, and it's abnormal again, a different way. I'm having an abortion on Thursday." My mother cried.

Dean's parents we wouldn't call until after the abortion, when we would tell them we had lost another pregnancy; and rather than risk a confrontation over moral issues, we would tell them I had miscarried.

A trip to the hospital on Wednesday to fill out admissions forms was just one more wearying event, an unwaivable bureaucratic requirement.

"If they ask," Dr. Barrie warned me over the phone, "don't mention you've been sick. As long as you don't have a fever now."

"I don't."

"Good, then we can get this over with tomorrow."

From the hospital, Dean drove me to Dr. Barrie's office for a preabortion procedure. Here I learned another peculiar word: laminaria. Seaweed, that's what it was. Sticks of it. Dr. Barrie was going to insert sticks of it into the opening of my cervix, where the sticks would expand overnight, absorbing fluid from my body, widening the opening, making the abortion easier, less painful. The box lay on the sink cabinet in the examining room. *Product of Japan*, it said. "Here's what they look like," Dr. Barrie said, holding up a thin brown dried stick the length of an extra-long cigarette. Like a Tampax, it had a string attached.

"Is this going to hurt?"

"It shouldn't be too bad."

A nurse stood by, handing Dr. Barrie what she needed—cotton swabs, tongs, the brown sticks. I lay there trying not to think too hard. Another ending.

Dr. Barrie worked the first stick of laminaria into the opening of my womb. The pain of it made me howl. Had she known how much it would hurt? Then she inserted the second stick, still more painful than the first. I started to cry, overwhelmed suddenly with pity for myself.

"I'll forget the third one," Dr. Barrie said.

That afternoon and evening, I was still pregnant, technically, but with the laminaria inside me the pregnancy was in a sense already over. Something irreversible had been done to the environment of the fetus. I couldn't forget that for a second. I just wanted it to be done with now. I kept thinking that once I wasn't pregnant anymore I could curl up on the bed for a few days and remember who I was.

When I woke up the next morning, the swollen laminaria were pressing painfully on my bladder and vagina. Peeing didn't help, and the pressure increased steadily during the drive to the hospital. At Brigham and Women's, the nurse assured me that the pressure I felt was a normal effect of the laminaria. "Your doctor should be here any minute. You can have her take the laminaria out right away."

While Dean waited in the hall, I went into a room with lockers and wooden benches, the sort of room we had in high school for changing into our gymsuits. At the far end of the room was a closetlike cubicle with a bench in it. I closed the door of the cubicle behind me and changed into one of the pale blue hospital johnnies, clean and neatly folded, piled on a shelf above the bench. Blue slippers, the spongy rubber kind I had used when I was hospitalized, were stacked in plastic bags on the shelf beside the johnnies. I stepped out of my sandals and put on a pair of slippers, then scooped my clothes off the bench. Next to me was a big rollaway barrel half-filled with johnnies; DEPOSIT USED JOHNNIES HERE said a sign on the wall above it, with an arrow pointing down. That would be for later. I went out to the lockers.

Three women were being escorted into the locker room by the supervising nurse who was giving them the same instructions she had given me. I looked away from them and found an empty locker for my clothes and went out into the hall to sit with Dean.

When Dr. Barrie arrived, her familiar, knowing, rising and falling "hi" helped give me courage. "They won't allow you in the room during the procedure," she told Dean.

I kissed and hugged him good-bye. "I'll be sitting right here in the hall," he said.

"It's such a depressing place for you to wait."

"Don't worry, I don't mind."

A nurse led me into a room with four beds—narrow stretcher-type beds on wheels—and instructed me to lie down on the one nearest the door. On the bed farthest from me, by the window, lay a woman with an IV tube attached to her arm. A nurse stood beside her adjusting the tube, speaking softly. "Just something to relax you," my nurse was saying to me as she jabbed an IV needle into the underside of my forearm. The nurse had short blond hair and her lips seemed constantly about to part in a smile. She made me feel safe. I tried to concentrate on her movements and on the murmur from the other bed. I looked forward to Dr. Barrie's pulling out the laminaria, relieving the pressure.

After several minutes, the nurse helped me off the stretcher and into an adjoining room, where I lay down again, this time with Dr. Barrie seated on a low stool at my feet. Dr. Barrie had me "scoot down" and place my slippered feet in the stirrups. I felt the discomfort of the speculum holding open my vagina, then Dr. Barrie easing the laminaria out of me. The pressure inside subsided.

"I'm going to give you a shot of novocaine in the cervix now," Dr. Barrie said. "It will help you." The nurse offered me her hand to hold. I gripped it.

"Didn't the laminaria help?"

"Yes, somewhat, but I'm afraid we still need the shot."

The jab hurt, but only a little. I pictured my cervix as something dark and soft like the meat of a snail. I imagined the fleshy opening forced apart just a pencil width or two, a reluctant mouth; I wanted to believe that the laminaria had done some good.

"This shouldn't hurt too much now," Dr. Barrie told me. "I'm going to begin the suction." A loud, rhythmic sucking sound came from a machine near the foot of the table. I tightened my grip on the nurse's hand. Something probed inside me, uncomfortable, making me twist my body. "It's important that you lie still," Dr. Barrie cautioned. Two or three minutes passed. The sound of the vacuum. The pain. The suppressed urge to move. Then, "That's all, now. It's over."

It's over. I had had my eyes clenched against the pain and the possibility of something going wrong. *It's over.* I opened my eyes and saw the nurse looking at me. My hand, I realized, was still clenched around hers. Slowly, I uncurled my fingers, and she gently withdrew her hand from mine.

Dr. Barrie removed her rubber gloves and came to stand beside me, and I could tell she would be leaving. I didn't want her to go. "Thank you," I said, "thank you for doing it yourself."

"It went well. You should be fine. But you must call if you have excessive bleeding or cramping or run a fever. The nurse will give you instructions. And I'll need to see you in two or three weeks. You should make an appointment. I'll let Dean know you're okay."

The nurse removed the IV needle from my arm and led me back to the bed in the next room. She put a sanitary pad between my legs. "I'd like you to rest here awhile. Just to be sure you're feeling okay. How are you doing?"

I started to cry.

"Do you want to talk?"

"I'm just sad."

The nurse looked at me, nodding, saying nothing. Finally, "Why don't you close your eyes and rest for a few minutes?" I followed her advice. I could hear her walk away and some other people come into the room.

I opened my eyes halfway to see a nurse leading a patient to the bed by the window. I closed my eyes again and let myself cry silently. I was grateful not to have to move. I kept wishing Dean were permitted in the room. I wanted to hold on to him. I wondered about the other patient. Was she like me? Had she wanted her baby? Was her husband waiting in the hall? Did she have a husband? I felt sorry for both of us.

"How're you doing?"

I opened my eyes to see the nurse smiling. I felt safe in that room, not eager to get up. The nurse raised my hospital johnny and checked the pad. "You're doing fine," she said. "Do you feel well enough to sit up? I have some information for you to read." She helped me into a sitting position and handed me a sheet of paper: WHAT TO DO AND WHAT TO EXPECT AFTER YOU HAVE AN ABORTION OR MISCARRIAGE. There were ten numbered paragraphs. The last one said: "REMEMBER: Call the doctor if you have any of the following: 1) fever of more than 100.4; 2) severe, persistent pain; 3) excessive bleeding." I turned the paper over. On the back were the same ten paragraphs, but in Spanish.

"Do you have any questions about anything mentioned on the sheet? Or is there anything else you want to ask me?"

"Do you think I'll be able to go back to work on Monday?"

"If you don't have any of these problems, yes, I would say so. But you should let your doctor know your plans, and you should pay attention to how tired you feel."

She helped me off the table. "How do you feel? Not dizzy?"

"I'll be okay. Thank you for your help. You've been very kind."

Out in the hall, Dean and I embraced.

When I went into the locker room to get changed, the three women were still there, all of them dressed now in the blue johnnies, sitting on the benches, talking. Again we said nothing to each other, but they were watching me as I opened my locker and took out my clothes, and finally I looked around at one of them. "How was it?" she said. "Did it hurt a lot?"

Her fear surprised me. I must have been assuming she'd been through this before. I was glad to be able to reassure her.

"It wasn't too bad really. It's very fast."

Somehow I found myself telling the three women how much I had wanted my baby.

"That's real sad," one of them said. The three of them nodded and clucked.

I wanted their sympathy, yes, but also, in sharing my plight with them, I wanted to accuse them. I had the impression, rightly or wrongly, that they were aborting unwanted, normal pregnancies. I pitied them, didn't wish to judge them, believed deeply in their right to choose to have an abortion; and yet I resented them. They made me jealous by being able to have what I wanted; and they made me angry by throwing the gift away. To them, though, it was an unwanted gift; I understood that. Some of my resentment grew from the fear I had that the so-called right-to-lifers would succeed in their fight against abortion rights. Though I knew abortion opponents could be as uncompromising about abnormal pregnancies as about normal ones, I also believed it was the thousands of aborted normal pregnancies that most aroused people's sensibilities and created national support for the right-to-life crusaders. As neither Dean nor I would have kept struggling to have a child if we had had no means of aborting an abnormal fetus, I worried, really worried, about losing my right to have an abortion. The legal controversy had become a matter of direct personal concern to me and to Dean. No freedom had ever seemed more precious.

I wished the women good luck and went out to Dean.

2

What I remember most vividly about the first few days following the abortion isn't my depression but my surges of energy.

"I can't believe you!" Dean kept saying. "Where are you finding it?"

As his spirits went on dragging, I felt almost apologetic about my optimistic mood. "Is it hard for you to take?"

"Well, maybe a little."

"I'm just so relieved. And my head isn't clogged. That feeling I get when I'm pregnant, like there's cotton in my head—it's gone already. Besides, I'm looking ahead. I really believe we're going to have a child someday. If we just try enough times."

I was obsessed with thinking about the next pregnancy. And the next. And the next. As many as it would take to produce a child.

I had come up with a theory that guaranteed success. It went like this: You know you can get pregnant. Easily, in fact. You don't have to worry about that anymore. So even if you have many losses—three, or four, or five—you can keep trying, and eventually you'll succeed. You're a realist now; you know you may have to go through this several times before you have a child. Next time you'll be more prepared.

I compared myself to women of my grandmother's generation, before the days of sophisticated medicine, when pregnancy loss, and even death in childbirth,

was more common. You don't need any extraordinary
courage, I told myself, just the kind of courage all
women used to have.

It was a book of memoirs by the novelist Eudora
Welty that started me thinking about women in the old
days. Knowing how I loved writers' autobiographies,
Dean had given me the book as a cheerer-upper a few
days before the abortion. I had been too distracted to
finish it but got far enough to read Welty's account of
how her mother had nearly died around the turn of the
century after giving birth to her first child, stillborn;
though dependent on the care of a country doctor
attending her at home, she had tried again. Reading
about her, I felt gutsier, and less inclined to pity myself. And less alone.

But Dean wasn't ready to share my view. He wasn't
sure he wanted to keep trying. He warned me, as he
had after Amelia died, that he might not want to risk
another loss. "Don't press me," he said once again, "I
need time to figure it out."

I knew we had solved this problem when we had
had it before. And I knew it was part of a pattern—me,
the impatient one, ready to plunge ahead; Dean, hesitant, creeping up on things, then suddenly decisive.

But I was frightened nonetheless. The one possibility
I couldn't fathom was giving up.

"Try to meet somewhere in the middle," our social
worker suggested. "Dean, you need to allow some
discussion of the subject, so Marion won't be so anxious, and you need to show an open mind. Marion,
you need to admit that Dean's fears are understandable
and that you share them too."

The gap between us was a painful contrast to our
closeness during my pregnancies when I was so vulnerable and Dean so protective. "It's hard taking care
of someone else," Dr. Barrie commented, "and Dean is
so good at it. Give him time, he'll come around."

Looking back now, the only wonder is that he came around so soon.

By October, three months after the abortion, Dean wanted to try again. By the end of November, I was pregnant, though I didn't suspect it until mid-December. I waited until the day before Christmas to go for a blood test, and on Christmas day I couldn't get a result because the lab was closed. I was glad it was closed—my hope was safe for the holiday.

The day after Christmas, I called Dr. Barrie. "Yes, you're pregnant," she said, "and your beta-sub is excellent this time, exactly what it should be."

That Friday, two days later, she examined me. "Relax," she told me. "You're fine. Your uterus is nicely expanded for six weeks, and I don't feel any fibroids."

She began thinking ahead. "Since Yale wants you to have an amniocentesis as a double check on the biopsy, we ought to set up a sixteen-week appointment for your amniocentesis. We should set up a twelve-week appointment with the nurse for a physical, too."

"I can't let myself think that far ahead. I'd like to wait until we have the results from Yale."

"I really think we should get you scheduled now."

Don't do it, I thought. "What if I wind up having to cancel the appointments again like last time? It just made me feel worse."

"I won't insist, but these appointments are hard to get, especially for the amniocentesis, so you should take care of this as soon as we get a result from the biopsy." Dr. Barrie paused. "You know, at some point you'll have to let yourself start thinking of your pregnancy as normal."

"I know." I sounded sheepish. "It seems impossible to me now. Maybe later I'll be able to."

Dr. Barrie picked up the little circular chart on her desk. I knew what it was, and I wanted to stop her, but I didn't. "Your due date is August 21."

Afterward, I pretended to myself that I hadn't heard

the number, just the month. But the following summer, when Dean's new secretary gave birth to a baby
boy on August 21, I stopped pretending and told Dean
about our due date. "It's just a date, he said, "like any
other. It was never really ours." He sincerely believed
that, but I didn't. To me it wasn't "just a date," and it
still isn't, even now.

After my exam, the only date I permitted myself to
think about was January 25, the date the biopsy was
scheduled at Yale. Dean and I had already booked a
room at the Colony Inn for the night before.

I opened *A Child Is Born* and searched for a picture of
a one-month-old embryo. *That's what it looks like now.*
Then I searched for a picture of a two-month-old fetus.
That's what it will be like when I got to Yale. I paid special
attention to the feathery villi.

So far, nothing had gone wrong. Last time, there
had been scares from the very beginning. This time
things were different. I paged through the book, even
looking at the later pictures, the ones that ought to
have been taboo.

I had a new niece by then. My sister-in-law had
given birth on October 3, my father's birthday. When
she called me from the hospital I didn't really want to
hear how she and the baby were doing. Instead of
feeling connected to the baby, as I had when my nephew
was born, I felt cut off. And I cut myself off. I refused
to look at pictures of my niece. When an envelope of
snapshots arrived in the mail, I had Dean look at them
for me and hide them in a drawer. When my mother
called, I didn't congratulate her, didn't say a word
about the baby. I resented my niece's existence, took
no pleasure in it. I didn't send any gift when she was
born, and at Christmas, when I ordered her a panda
bear out of a catalog, it certainly wasn't love for the
baby that prompted me.

Around the time my niece was born, I received a flier in the mail from a babies' furniture company. I was used to getting that kind of mail, it had been arriving for over a year. I had become fairly inured to it, and so had Dean. I always threw such mail out before Dean could see it, and (as he recently told me) if he found it first, he did the same for me.

But this particular ad I remember because it might have been glued to my hand, the way I kept holding it, reading and rereading it, unable to throw it out, finally letting myself sit down and cry. It was the two words at the top in bold print that got to me: FIRST BIRTHDAY.

Dean was working hard that fall, and by Christmas he was exhausted and unhappy with his job. He took a week off just to rest at home, and to make it seem more like a vacation, we spent the weekend before New Year's at a new hotel in Boston on Copley Square. It was a novelty for us to be going into Boston to stay at a hotel, like a couple of tourists; but the even greater novelty that weekend was the weather. Huge blocks of ice that had been trucked into the square to be carved into sculptures for Boston's "First Night" celebration were melting under the sculptors' hands. The temperature was in the seventies. It felt as though by some error a remnant of summer had never been discarded and we had discovered it and wrapped it around us, Dean and I and all the other people standing outside looking at each other with incredulous smiles. Don't be fooled, we had to tell ourselves, it won't last.

As I think of it now, my pregnancy was the same way.

In our hotel room at night, on the thirtieth floor, we turned our armchairs to face the wall of windows and sat talking, looking out over a panorama of the Charles and Cambridge and the towns farther out. We tried to identify things: the buildings in Cambridge; the major roads, where strings of lights moved; the dark ring of

hills at the horizon. Sitting there together, it was hard
not to feel optimistic.

"You know that picture of my brother's kids?" Dean
asked.

"Yup," I said. In my mind, I could see the two little
girls and the boy, he just a couple of months older than
Amelia would have been, the three of them perched in
a row on a brick step in front of a fireplace, their feet
flat on the carpet below the step, their knees the height
of their chests. Little Johnny was blond and fair-skinned
and delicate.

"Those are cute kids, aren't they?"

"Yup, they sure are."

"I was thinking, maybe this time it's gonna work
out. I'd like to be a father . . . you know?"

"I know."

I imagined a phone call—the same one I had imagined during my second pregnancy. I was calling my
parents, telling them I was pregnant and had been to
Yale and knew the baby was going to be all right. Did
Dean, I wondered, rehearse a similar phone call to his
parents? I never asked him; there were limits to what
we could bear to say to each other, and bear to hear
each other say.

During my second pregnancy, three of my friends
had said they "had a good feeling this time." Now, the
third time, they didn't make predictions. But this time
things did seem to be going well, and Dean and I had,
beneath the tight skin of realism that covered our
thoughts, a hope that was more like a prayer.

On Monday, January 14, eleven days before I was
scheduled to go to Yale, I drove myself to Dr. Abram's
office for an ultrasound exam. Dean had offered to meet
me there, but I felt confident enough to go alone. "It's
silly for you to bother," I told him. "I'll only be there
a few minutes, and everything's going fine this time."

I drove with a thermos of apple juice beside me, and at red lights I forced myself to drink. By now, I knew just how much to drink, and how fast, so that my bladder would be full for the exam at Dr. Abram's but not so full that I couldn't hold it in.

"My bladder's full," I told the receptionist.

"She'll be right with you."

"Marion Wasserman?" Dr. Abram's assistant appeared in the waiting room, and I followed her down the hall.

I lay on the examining table and watched the speckly gray patterns on the screen. "I'll just get you started here." Dr. Abram's assistant pressed the sensor against my belly. I wondered if I would be able to see the heartbeat.

"I'm not getting an image."

"What do you mean?"

"I don't know why, but I don't see the embryo. I'm just having trouble for some reason. I think I'll put you in the other examining room. The equipment in there is a little different. Dr. Abram should be able to get a picture."

She doesn't really believe that, said a voice inside me I didn't want to hear, she's giving up too soon. You're just nervous, said another voice.

In the other room I lay down again, and the assistant switched on the screen. When Dr. Abram came in, I wanted to be sure she remembered me: "I'll be going to Yale again. You remember, right? For the villus biopsy. I'm here to be sure everything's okay before I go."

She smiled and nodded, leaning over me to press the sensor against my belly. As she looked at the screen, past my shoulder, where I couldn't see it, her face was expressionless.

I grabbed her bare forearm and held it. "Is something wrong? I'm getting the feeling something's wrong."

She looked at me and smiled again. "Nothing's wrong."

I loosened my grip on her arm.

"I'm just nervous," I apologized. "I've been through so much."

"I know you have." Dr. Abram adjusted something on the machine, then began pressing against my abdomen again.

"There's no fetus here."

"What?"

"There's no fetus here. This happens sometimes. It's not uncommon. The embryo doesn't develop and you miscarry."

"You mean it's not good?" *It's got to be.* "It's really not good again? How can you be sure?"

"I'm sure. There's no fetus here. You'll miscarry."

I started to cry.

"It'll work for you eventually, I know it will. I've seen women go through this four or five times. Some day I'll see you here with a healthy pregnancy. You can't believe that now, but it's true."

"I'm already thirty-six."

"That's young. One of my patients is forty-three and just had her first baby."

I don't want my first baby at forty-three. I want this baby. There is no this baby.

"I'm going to call Dr. Barrie and tell her. If you want to speak to her too, you can call her on my phone. But take your time. Lie there a few minutes."

Dr. Abram left the room, shutting the door. I could hear women's voices in the hall. I sat up and raised my hand in the air in a fist and smashed it down against the table.

I was afraid to move, to stand up, to open the door.

On the phone, Dr. Barrie explained to me that Dr. Abram was not in any doubt—she was certain there was no fetus. No one could be sure why this had happened, but this was nature's way of eliminating an embryo that wasn't developing properly, perhaps an embryo that from the first stages had divided into the wrong number of cells.

"When will it come?"

"It could happen very soon, or it could take a while. I think we should schedule a D & C. That will be easier on you."

"You mean like last time?"

"The same."

"At the hospital?"

"Yes. Just the same."

"Will you do it for me again?"

"Yes, of course."

"This your first?" I was sitting in the reception area of Dr. Abram's office, incapable of driving myself home, waiting for Dean. A gray-haired woman was chatting with the woman next to her, visibly pregnant.

"My second."

"What are you hoping for?"

"A boy, definitely a boy. It would be nice if you could choose, wouldn't it?"

I left the office and stood in the stairwell, staring out a window at the courtyard. The dull gray light was just beginning to fade.

"She called it a blighted ovum." I turned and saw a couple coming down the stairs from the landing outside the doctor's office, holding hands. "She says it's stopped developing," the woman was saying. "I'm going to miscarry."

Blighted ovum. The phrase brought to mind something round and bleached. Something small and waxy, the size of a pea. Blighted ovum. Dr. Abram hadn't used that phrase with me, but it fit.

A gust of cold air filled the stairwell as the man pulled open the street door. The woman looked at me. I imagined myself saying something to her—some word of sympathy; I wanted to give her something for making me feel less alone. I remember being surprised by the calmness of her features. It must be her first time, I thought, she's explained it away already. She's ready to try again. She still has faith.

And then Dean was there in the courtyard, walking fast toward the door, his briefcase in hand, his knit cap pulled down over his ears. I ran out to him and we hugged each other as tight as it was possible to hug; then we sat on one of the cement benches and held each other some more. I didn't care that it was cold. I didn't want to go home.

The next morning, I scheduled the D & C for Friday, four days away. There were no earlier openings, and because of my new job I was actually glad. Since September, I had been teaching writing at Tufts, no longer practicing law. With a Friday appointment, I would be able to teach my first class of the winter term, on Thursday, and after resting over the weekend, return to teaching on Monday. All without skipping a beat.

I had a feeling that I had seemed tired, depressed first semester. How could my students not have noticed? I had had to struggle to find the energy for the smallest exertions, and had often failed. The five-minute walk from my office to the classroom had seemed like miles; I would think of carrying an extra book to class to read a special passage to the students, but the thought of the added weight in my briefcase would be enough to make me leave the book on my desk. I was determined to be more normal this semester, not to let my private troubles drag at me in the classroom. Having failed to become a mother, and having abandoned law, it seemed doubly important that I not disappoint myself in my teaching. For my new set of students, I would wear a happier face. It wasn't going to be easy.

The D & C would be done in the outpatient department of Brigham and Women's. The unit I had been in before—where every patient was ending a pregnancy, and the nurses were used to caring for women in my predicament—had no time available until the following week. I wanted to get the procedure over with; and besides, my body might not wait a whole week.

"What happens if it just starts to come?" I had asked Dr. Barrie. "Will it hurt?"

She had explained that I would probably feel some cramping, and that the bleeding could get messy. "I would much rather have you get this done before that happens," she had said. "If you do start to miscarry, save any large pieces of tissue, and call me right away."

I convinced myself that my body would wait until Friday.

"Why don't you get someone to take over your class?" a friend of mine asked. "Why push yourself?"

But I did push myself. And even if I hadn't, my body still might not have waited.

On Wednesday, I had to go through the Brigham and Women's admitting procedure, as I had in July, before my abortion. "They won't let you out of it," the assistant at my health center told me. The proverbial salt on the wound.

After being examined by Dr. Barrie (who told me my uterus was smaller than it had been at six weeks), I drove to the hospital and proceeded through several hours of waiting—to give blood and urine samples; to be given a plastic ID card; to be given a second card after a nurse lost the first; to be interviewed by an anesthesiologist who, in spite of my insistence that I wouldn't be having general anesthesia, gave me a run-down of the "options" I ought to consider, until I was so scared and perplexed I called Dr. Barrie for reassurance.

"No general anesthesia," she told me. "Don't worry, they don't give you anything I don't order."

Forcing myself through the hospital routine, I felt oddly removed from what I was doing, almost like a sleep-walker. It was only that anesthesiologist who cracked my control; with him, I had to fight hard not to cry.

I recognized the pinched-faced woman at the lab; she had been there over a year before, when I had been admitted for surgery. "Have a seat," she said without looking up, taking my papers from me, shoving them into a tray on her cluttered desk. I thought back to the fear I had had when I was being admitted for surgery. At least this wasn't surgery; no knife, no general anesthesia, no overnight stay.

From one of the two doors marked *Lavatory*, an elderly man emerged carrying a vial of yellow fluid. He steadied himself for a moment against the curved wall. The circular, windowless waiting area, though on the main floor of the hospital, had a subterranean closeness and gloom.

The receptionist's arm looped like a tentacle towards the tray of papers. "O'Connor," she said without turning her head towards the patients and without raising her voice. "O'Connor," she repeated.

A young woman sitting near me pushed herself slowly up out of her chair. Her huge belly dragged on my attention like a magnet, and other patients were staring at it too. It was almost as though you could see the baby she had in there.

I'm pregnant, too, I was thinking. Or am I? If you have a blighted ovum, are you pregnant?

I watched the woman enter the lavatory; pictured her on the toilet with her big belly. I wondered what it would be like to be her—getting admitted to give birth.

The next afternoon, climbing the long flight of stone steps at Tufts's main gate, I felt crampy and tired and found myself actually tempted to sit down right there on the cold steps. I was heading to my office on the quadrangle at the top of the hill to run off a syllabus for my class. Winter was like winter now; I kept clutching the hood of my coat under my chin to keep it from blowing back off my head. Each step, as I slowly alternated my weight from one boot to the other, taking care to grip the metal railing and to avoid the patches of ice and snow, caused a strain that radiated through me from my abdomen. I wasn't sure if it meant anything. You're just being a worrier, I told myself.

In the office building, I ran off my syllabus and went to the Ladies Room. The pad I had put in my underpants—just in case—was bloody.

How bad would it get? How fast would it come? *I can't teach now. I can't possibly.*

I got Dr. Barrie on the phone and she told me to call Dean and have him drive me to Brigham and Women's for an emergency D & C. Dr. Barrie would alert Dr. O'Shea, who was on duty at the hospital.

"Hurry," I told Dean when I spoke to him at work. Even though Dr. Barrie had said there was no reason to panic, I was scared. It would take Dean probably forty minutes to get to Tufts by cab, and at least as much time to drive us to the hospital.

No one I worked with at Tufts knew I was pregnant, and even now, when I needed to ask for help, I was worried about letting too many people in on my problem. Fortunately, those colleagues I now confided in were ready to help: one took over my class for me; another offered to keep me company until Dean arrived, letting me sit with her in her office, where I was safe from conversation with anyone else. She had had pregnancy problems too. She understood.

At three-thirty, when she left to teach a class of her own, I began to worry about Dean. Where was he?

I walked down the hall to my office and saw the note my colleague had taped to the door telling Dean where to find me. The door was open and the note was facing into the room more than the hall. My office mate looked up. "Is something wrong?" He didn't know about my problem, and he was in the middle of a conference with a student.

"Has my husband been here looking for me?"

"There was someone about fifteen minutes ago. In a rush. Tall, blond."

Outside, snow was beginning to fall. Dean wasn't there. I'd rushed down the three flights of stairs, and now I was winded. For Christ's sake, I thought, why hadn't I realized that Dean might miss the note? For a moment, standing there in the snow without a coat on, I was paralyzed, too tired and cold to keep standing there, and at the same time afraid to climb back upstairs. Climb slowly, I told myself, while my mind raced.

"He's with the campus police," the department secretary told me. "He's pretty upset."

She placed a call to the police and in a few minutes I was in the police car with Dean, being taken to the spot where my car was parked. It was obvious to me that Dean would have been weeping if he weren't still, in spite of his ordeal, being brave for me. "I didn't have any idea where you were," he said. "No one knew. I thought maybe you'd been taken to the hospital. Another hospital, even. I was scared, I was so scared." As he drove us through rush hour traffic along the snowy streets into Boston, I kept apologizing. The panic I had caused him had been so terrible that I could feel it coming from him still, like smoke after a fire. Later that night, at home in bed, Dean told me again how scared he had been. Only this time he let himself weep.

At the emergency unit, Dean and I were directed off a circular corridor into a windowless room shaped like a pie wedge with the pointy end lopped off. I put on a hospital johnny and lay down on a padded table with stirrups. There was clean paper under me, and a pillow, and the nurse found a blanket to keep me warm. Curtains for pulling around the table were drawn to one side, and I took some comfort from their familiar fabric, the same as had been used for window curtains in my hospital rooms. The curtains and floor were stained with blood and iodine. Strange as it seems, I found the stains reassuring. Here things were expedited rather than fussed and worried over. In. Out. That was what I wanted. Get it done with. Get me home.

Two nurses introduced themselves. The older, more commanding of the two told me they would give me Valium intravenously to relax me. Though I normally resisted taking drugs, I wanted the Valium. I knew I needed to be made calmer. The day had been a nightmare.

The younger nurse pushed on the veins on the top side of my left hand. "Your veins are small," she said. No nurse had ever told me that before.

"Why are you doing it in my hand? They used my wrist the other times I was here."

The nurse gave me a dumb stare and jabbed the needle a second, then a third, time into the same hole; the spot burned as though the needle had been dipped in acid. I don't know how many times she would have jabbed me if I hadn't shrieked at her to stop. When she backed off, the older nurse inserted the needle easily into the vein at my right wrist. I should have told them no students, I thought, I don't need this.

The nurses left the room by an inner door that I assumed led to the central circle inside the pie. The room, heavily soundproofed, was quiet but for a whirring somewhere in the ceiling. Soon, the older nurse returned with Dr. O'Shea, who greeted Dean and me sympathetically. Then it was like the last time, but without a shot of novocaine; I heard a rhythmic motor and felt a nasty cramping. When it was over, the nurse and the doctor left me with Dean to "rest awhile."

"The needle hurts," I complained to Dean. "Can you tell them we just want to leave?" Dean knocked on the inner door and spoke to the nurse.

"She can't do anything without Dr. O'Shea," he reported. "She's going to call for her."

After five or ten minutes, I threatened to get up with the IV in (knowing I couldn't, because it was on a pole attached to the table). Dean knocked on the door again. "She'll get up herself," I heard him say. A few minutes later, Dr. O'Shea arrived, and the nurse untaped the needle.

While I put my clothes back on, I noticed the large spots of fresh blood on the floor by the foot of the table. That's what pregnancy was for me and Dean. Blood. Just blood. And pain. And nothing to show for it.

Loss, I discovered then, wasn't something you practiced. It wasn't something you got good at. My theorizing after my second pregnancy had been naive. I had assumed that loss after loss after loss my optimism would be there to push me along; I had actually assumed that a third loss would be easier than a second.

As it turned out, the opposite was true. Losing a third time was harder. The losses accumulated. A tangible weight was bearing me down, and it had increased now. I saw myself bent forward with a bulging sack slung over my shoulder, balanced on my back— ironically like a Santa. Each bulge in the sack was a child, or almost-child. Santa carried toys; he could set them down and oversee the opening of the gifts. What I carried I could never set down and never give away. And the burden had suddenly become leaden. I staggered under it, or stood still. Sometimes it made me weep unexpectedly.

I questioned—truly questioned—whether I would ever want to risk adding to the freight of losses I supported. Part of me wanted to try again; but part of me said, "No, don't ever do it. If the pregnancy doesn't succeed, you'll collapse under the weight."

If only I could take several years off, I thought. But I couldn't. I was going to be thirty-seven in April.

After three weeks, I received a phone call at home one evening from Dr. Barrie. The phone was ringing as I put my key in the door when I came home from work.

"Hi." When I heard Dr. Barrie's rising, falling greeting, I remembered that it was Wednesday and my appointment with her, for a post D & C checkup, was scheduled for Friday. She's calling to change the time, I thought, but then, just as I began to wonder why she hadn't delegated the call to her secretary, she said something strange, something that made me sit down in the kitchen chair with my coat still on, as though someone had shoved me there. "We received the pathology report on the placenta. It's abnormal."

What now? What's she telling me?

"You had what we call a partial molar pregnancy. This is a disease of the placental tissue that can be malignant in some cases, but I've talked with the pathologist, and he's not worried about your case. It's the most benign form."

I had to strain to keep hearing Dr. Barrie's voice. I've got cancer, I thought. Some mild form, but cancer. "Most benign." That means least malignant.

"We need to have your blood tested every week until your beta-sub has been zero for three weeks. Then, we need a test every month for a total of six months. You'll be fine. I'm not worried. Even the more serious molar pregnancies I've seen were cured. It just takes a while. And I must ask you not to get pregnant for one year."

"Pregnant! That's no problem. This is it. I'm through trying. I don't want to get pregnant any more."

"Well, you needn't decide that now."

I heard Dean at the door. He came into the kitchen,

and I knew he could see right away that something was wrong. "It's Dr. Barrie," I said, leaning my head on my hand and looking up at him, while I tried to pay attention to the doctor's faraway voice.

"I can explain more to you when I see you Friday," she was saying.

"What is it? What's wrong?" Dean was asking. "Let me in on it."

"Will you just explain this to Dean a minute? He just walked in, and he's going crazy here wondering what we're talking about."

Dean took the phone and heard what I had heard. When he hung up, I began crying. I was terrified.

"I don't think you have cancer," Dean told me. "I think you misunderstood."

But why had Dr. Barrie said "most benign" and not "benign"? And why did she want me to go for a chest X ray? "Just routine," she had said. "It will be negative, but it's routine in these cases. When the cells are malignant, they sometimes appear in the lungs."

I kept waking during the night. And the next evening, driving home from work, my conviction that I had cancer fed mercilessly upon itself, so that I wept as I drove.

On Friday, at the health center, I asked Dean to speak to Dr. Barrie first, alone, to discover whether I did or did not have cancer. Dean had gone to a bookstore the day before and had read about molar pregnancies and he had concluded that the type I had was not malignant. Now, he walked toward me in the lounge after speaking with the doctor, and I was exquisitely afraid to hear what he would say.

"It's okay, you misunderstood. It's definitely not cancer."

And then Dr. Barrie showed us pictures of molar tissue. The spectrum of types: benign, with barely detectable pockets or "moles"; and cancerous, with large grapelike moles. "Molar pregnancies are rare," Dr. Barrie said. "Only one in roughly two thousand pregnancies are molar. Once it occurs, you're at a considerably higher risk of having another molar pregnancy. On the other hand, I know a doctor who had a very serious molar pregnancy. She adopted a child afterwards but then later had a normal pregnancy. You needn't rule out another pregnancy."

"Yes, but with the genetic problem, too. It seems crazy. There are too many obstacles. Pregnancy for me has gotten to be insane. Look at me, I'm a wreck."

"Well, you may decide against it. But in any case, I'd want you to wait a year, so you needn't decide now."

"What happens if I get pregnant while I've got this condition?"

"You won't ovulate or get a period until it clears up, so you can't get pregnant. But even after your beta-sub returns to zero you're going to continue with the blood tests until you've had six months of negative tests. If you got pregnant during that time, we couldn't judge the beta-sub results. We wouldn't be able to get the six months of negative tests necessary to assure us you've recovered."

"Why did you say I should wait a whole year?"

"That's what we advise. I've had patients who just won't wait, though. After the six months, they . . ."

"Well, none of it matters for me. I'm through getting pregnant." It amazed me when I said those words that I knew I meant them. I wasn't just begging for sympathy or reassurance or a protest from Dean. I meant them. The last thing I wanted was for Dean or Dr. Barrie or anyone else to try to talk me into another pregnancy. My determination to have a child had finally collapsed, crumbled, blown away.

"We're planning a trip to Europe in June. We'll be gone three weeks. This will be the first summer in three years that will center on something wonderful and exciting instead of our latest messed-up pregnancy.

These blood tests won't prevent us from going, will they?"

"Well, I would like you to have a zero, or near zero, beta-sub before you go. I think you will, by then, so it should work out. But let's wait a few weeks to see how fast the count is dropping."

Technically, because of the diseased cells, my body thought I was pregnant. My body was producing hormones appropriate to the early weeks after conception. How ironic it all was. After three losses, and with my knowing, finally, that I would never try again, my body refused to accept the message that I was no longer pregnant. Like someone going through a slow divorce, I was forced to deal with details of a life that was over. Each time I went for a blood test, I felt myself still caught within the chain of medical revelations that had begun with my first conception, over two years in the past. Almost without fail, a visibly pregnant woman waited near me in one of the lounge chairs at the lab, or a new parent sat there caressing an infant. And I remembered that first blood test when they had asked me for a fresh sample of urine and I had felt so impatient, so eager, for the results.

As my beta-sub count decreased, in a geometric progression, approximately halved each week, I became more and more willing to believe that this latest worry would soon come to an end. It was still difficult for me to imagine a routine not focused on blood. But I began to recall that I had once lived such a life; and now I longed to have it back.

CHAPTER 7

OUT OF
THE BATTLE

"I'll be driving along—it happens all the time on my
way to work—and I'm slowing down, not even seeing
the road, staring off to the side, the sidewalk. Yesterday, there was a father and his little boy. It's like I've
never noticed people before, never really looked. This
man and his kid, they both had glasses and blond hair,
straight as straw, real light blond. And they were short
and stocky, the two of them, with these funny little
owl noses, pointy little beaks. So damned alike! That's
all I can think: they're so alike, and they just accept it,
they don't even know how amazing it is. I look at them
so closely, it's like I'm on the sidewalk next to them,
not in my car—yet my hands are gripping the wheel
hard, and common sense is telling me, watch the road.
Yesterday, for the first time, I actually had to pull
over."

"What kinds of people do you look at?" my social
worker asks.

"It's these pairs, fathers and sons, mothers and daugh-
ters. The key thing is they look alike. There doesn't
even have to be a little kid—there might be a woman
my mother's age with a daughter my age. What I'm
obsessed with is the genes, the way the connection is

169

written in the stoop of a child's back, or the shape of his brows—that's what makes the staring different this time. Pregnant women still bother me too, of course. I stare at them. And little girls who look the way I picture Amelia—they make me feel so bad I want to look away, but instead I stare."

"Tell me again how you picture Amelia."

"Like me, like I was as a little girl—wavy brown hair, green eyes; mischievous, pretty. That's how I picture Amelia. But then I always wonder, maybe she would have been like Dean: blond, pale-skinned, maybe even a redhead. Dean's father's hair is reddish, and Dean has that color in his mustache. I feel so cheated because I'll never know."

"What does it feel like when you look at these other people?"

"They're not really people to me. More like props. Objects. I've never been a kleptomaniac, but I get this kind of rush when I'm staring, a physical excitement; my breathing gets tight. I bet kleptos feel like that before they steal something."

"What is it you want from these people?"

"What is it I want?"

I close my eyes and think, repeating the question to myself. What is it I want from all these strangers? What is it I want?

"I want to be them," I tell the social worker finally. "That's what it is. I want to be them. I want to climb inside them and have what they have."

After that conversation, I stared at other people less and less. After all, what was the point of staring? They could never give me what I wanted, I understood that now.

But the alternative to studying them was to look at myself—to accept my body, my future. And these seemed empty.

My fantasy child was gone. Where there had once

been conversation, there was silence. Not just the silence I had lived with since Amelia's death, when I
began refusing to hear that inner voice. Now the fantasy itself was dead, there was no voice. Sometimes I
noticed this, and I felt sickened, the way you feel when
you look at a stranger with some piece missing, an eye
or a hand.

There was a numbness too. The world and I didn't
have the same relationship we used to. The creating
and interweaving of life made me turn away, like an
intruder. My brother, my cousins, they spun life out of
themselves like the colored scarves of a magician. But
me, I was a tag end, a false lead. When I pictured the
family tree, my name was stuck out to the side, nothing flowing from it.

Reminders of my differentness were everywhere. Nov-
els and movies hurt when they dwelled on family re-
semblances and continuity, which I noticed they almost
always did—it was the great theme of life. That spring,
the greening of the world—the renewal I had felt so
intimately a part of two springs before—made me feel
abnormal, outside of nature. And that August, when
our pair of "pet" cardinals appeared at our birdfeeder
with a pumpkin-colored fledgling, my natural joy at
such a sight was mixed with jealousy. Imagine! Jealous
of a mother bird!

Sex seemed different too. Never again would Dean
and I make love with the intention of producing a
child. We had to use a condom or a diaphragm now,
and it would always be that way. For months after my
miscarriage I couldn't enjoy sex. It just made me feel
sad, depressed.

"You got laid for years without it having anything to
do with making a baby," Dean said. "Don't you remember? You liked it then."

"I know, but I can't seem to remember how to feel
that way anymore."

"I'll help you remember."

*   *   *

Still, in spite of these feelings, I clung to my decision never to get pregnant again.

I was like a wounded soldier home from the front. I wasn't victorious, and life wasn't normal, but it was a relief to be out of the battle.

In my relief, however, I suspected myself of cowardice. For weeks after Dr. Barrie called me, I kept asking myself if I should have had the courage at least to keep the question open, since I wasn't supposed to get pregnant anyway for another year. Was it wrong of me, I wondered, to want to be absolutely free of the struggle once and for all? Dr. Barrie hadn't quite said that it would be crazy for me to risk another molar pregnancy, so why did it seem crazy to me?

When I asked Dean what he thought, he said I had "51 percent of the vote" because it was my body on the line; he said my "no" was good enough for him.

"But what do *you* want?" I asked.

"I don't know what I'd say if you wanted to keep trying. I might say no."

I didn't know what or who I needed to put my mind at rest about my decision, but I knew I needed more than just time. I needed something that I couldn't find by myself, and that Dean and Dr. Barrie couldn't give me.

It was in May, a few weeks before Dean and I left for Europe (I had finally gotten my period by then, and Dr. Barrie had given our vacation her approval), that my family doctor conveyed to me, through Dr. Barrie, a general offer of sympathy and counsel.

I liked my family doctor. She was about my age, with my coloring; less easily alarmed than I, rather like Dean in the way she projected security. She was utterly without pretension, the only one of my doctors whom I thought of by her first name (though still, I didn't call her by it). And there was something about her—something difficult to pinpoint—that made her appealingly goofy. Something about her scratchy voice, about the way her eyes and brows were set close to her nose, about the way her mouth seemed stuck on at a slant. And I always had the feeling that she was laughing inside, laughing out of sympathy, laughing at the great cosmic joke played on all of us.

It was only after I went to see her that I stopped second-guessing my decision.

I sat down in her office, ready to review the medical details she was unfamiliar with and to hear what she thought about my risking another molar pregnancy. But she surprised me. She said my focus was wrong, I was asking the wrong questions.

"I don't know what the statistics are on molar pregnancies," she said, "Dr. Barrie can tell you that. But my guess is that you still have roughly a 25 percent chance of something going wrong, just as you did before your last pregnancy. I don't think the risks, overall, have increased significantly, but why do you care? That's not the issue you should be thinking about. What matters is what you and Dean believe another pregnancy would be like for you. That's what should guide you, not the textbook view of this or that complication."

She and I talked for two hours. I remember another doctor knocking on her door and asking if she would be going to lunch. She motioned him away.

She wanted to hear what Dean and I had been through, not medically, but emotionally. She asked questions I never would have expected from a doctor. What did the baby look like when you held her? How big was she? What color was her skin? Did Dean have friends he could turn to while you were in the hospital? How has your work life been affected? If you get pregnant again, what will your fears be? Will they begin right away? Will they let up after you go to Yale? After amniocentesis? When? And what is it you're so afraid of missing? Assuming you can adopt a child, what is it that makes it so important to go through a pregnancy?

I worked hard giving an answer to that last question, and the truth, when I spoke it, made me cry. I told her I wanted to participate in the miracle at the center of life—the bringing of being out of the void. I wanted the high of pregnancy: that feeling that carries one beyond oneself, pulls one into the mysterious circle of creation, merges the "I" with the "other."

"I know that the love I felt when I was pregnant was in part self-love, but it was also love for a new human being and love for the world and the way it all works. Being pregnant was a mystical experience at times. How can I stop myself from wanting that?"

My doctor closed her eyes tight for a moment, and I realized suddenly that she was holding back tears. Then she looked at me, and the laughter I always seemed to see in her eyes had been transmuted into a private pain. As she reached for a tissue, her thin mouth twisted into a half smile. "I don't do this," she said, "I just don't do this." She dabbed at the tears and blew her nose.

"Please." I hesitated; the patient wasn't supposed to be reassuring the doctor. "Please don't be embarrassed."

"I had pregnancy problems too," she said. "For years, and I thought about all these things you're saying."

"I had no idea." I sat there, shaking my head, thinking back to a day the summer before when I had seen my doctor from a distance. She had seemed to me to be the very ideal of the pregnant woman, truly transformed by her pregnancy into a more beautiful version of herself. I had felt so jealous, so resentful. I had assumed that for her it had been easy.

"I know the longing you're talking about," she said. "I used to try to make it go away."

"Did you ever think it was something you couldn't help, something built into you? You know, a sort of program designed to keep the species going?"

"Yes, I did. Is that what you think?"

"Yes, it is." I played with the soggy tissue in my hands, unconsciously tearing it into pieces until my lap and the carpet by my chair were dotted with ricelike shreds of paper. "Oh, God, look what I've done to your office."

"And that was the last tissue. We're out." My doctor laughed. She tilted the empty box on her desk so I could see into it. I laughed too, trying to roll the paper crumbs on my lap into one disposable ball.

"I think my biggest fear is that I'll be bitter for the rest of my life because I couldn't have this experience. I don't want to be bitter."

"Let me tell you about a couple I know. They're not patients of mine, they're friends. They've lost three times. Their first child was a daughter who died after living ten days, their second and third pregnancies both had fatal complications in the second trimester. They were so filled with grief that life seemed to come to a halt for them and they couldn't face another pregnancy. But they adopted a little girl, and in spite of everything life began moving forward for them again. They're not stuck anymore."

"Three losses? Just like us?"

"Three losses."

"I've been feeling like it was only us."

My doctor smiled, and for several seconds we just sat there contemplating each other.

"I can't tell you and Dean what to do . . ."

"I know."

". . . but I can think of no surer way for you to pick yourselves up and move on than to adopt. Before I finally gave birth to my son, I thought of adopting, and like you I didn't think it would be good enough, I was suspicious of it. Well, I know now that it would have been every bit as good, I'm sure of it. When I hold my son in my arms, I am absolutely convinced that the love I feel for him has nothing to do with my having delivered him. I often think that one of the mysteries about him is that it seems as though he just landed from the sky. He's his own little being, so separate, so complete. It's going to be such a wonder to see what he turns out to be, to watch him unfold in the coming years. All this would feel precisely the same with an adopted child. And remember, when that child turns to you, you're it's mother, it's not going to make any distinctions. I never get over how much my child needs me, how utterly helpless he is."

When I got up to leave, my doctor got up too. "I want to hug you," she said. We held each other tight, much more like friends than doctor and patient. "Good luck."

When I left her office, I had a new conviction about my decision. I knew that my relief was something good that I owed to myself, peaceful ground from which to look ahead and lay new plans. Whatever pregnancy may once have meant to me and Dean, it was time to put it behind us. It was only joyous in the abstract now; the reality was terrifying; and the cycle of losses and recoveries, if prolonged, might exhaust the years remaining to us in which to become parents.

CHAPTER 8

ACCEPTANCE

All along I had thought of adoption as something for other people, not for me and Dean. Second best, I had thought. It will never come to that.

Yet at the moment I decided against another pregnancy—on the phone that evening with Dr. Barrie—I knew (not on the surface of my thoughts, but deep down, in the part of me that simply refused to be cheated out of parenthood) that I would try adoption. Adoption was my safety net, the alternative that made giving up bearable. I couldn't begin to think of one without the other. Indeed, one of the advantages of making an absolute decision against another pregnancy was that Dean and I could concentrate completely on adoption.

After Amelia died—that summer before my surgery, when I was afraid I might require a hysterectomy—I had sent away to an adoption agency for an information package. I had never shown the information to Dean, or discussed it with him, and I had filed it away, convincing myself that I would never need it. Now, two years later, I pulled it out and reread it.

Just thinking of how long and frustrating the adoption process was likely to be made me weary; I was tired of facing obstacles, tired of having to be patient. But it was precisely my oppressive sense of so much time having passed without result that made me want

to hurry now—to identify a good adoption agency as
quickly as possible and apply for a child. When my
spirits sagged, it helped to remember that in this struggle my body—my health—would not be on the line. In
that sense, compared to what I had been through, it
would be easy.

Dean was not enthusiastic. When I talked to him
about adoption, he kept a barrier between us; we might
have been talking through one of those Plexiglass di-
viders taxi drivers use for protection.

Not that he had any objection to the idea of being an
adoptive parent—on the contrary, unlike me, he had
never viewed adoption as second best. His problem
was the same as it had been after our first two losses: a
hesitancy about trying to become a parent again; a fear
of disappointment.

Before we left for Europe, Dean and I turned to our
social worker for help. Dean had been asking me to put
the subject of adoption on hold until we returned from
our three-week trip, but I had refused to agree. As in
the past, our social worker suggested compromise. "Why
not agree that you'll only raise the issue if it's very
necessary? Who knows, Dean, once you get away, *you*
may want to discuss it."

After our trip, we continued seeing the social worker
on and off into the fall, talking to her about our different fears: Dean's of another losing effort, and mine of
not fully accepting a child I hadn't delivered. It was a
comfort to be discussing these issues with the same
therapist we had been seeing all along. Here was one
person we could absolutely trust to understand our
wariness.

While the counseling proceeded, I went ahead and
gathered information, making phone calls, writing let-
ters, reading books, even attending an introductory
lecture at an adoption agency. And in November Dean
agreed to visit two other agencies with me, and finally
to meet with the couple our doctor had told me about

who had had three losses and had adopted a little girl. Still, though, Dean insisted that he wasn't ready, might never be ready, to apply for a child.

One evening a few weeks before New Year's (it would soon be 1986, a year since my miscarriage, three years since Amelia's conception), I pressed Dean yet again, but there was no shattering the barrier between us. He continued to insist that he might choose to remain childless permanently. That night falling asleep next to him was impossible; I was so angry, my hands tightened into fists, and I kept imagining myself boxing him in the side. I got out of bed and went into our spare bedroom to sleep.

The next morning, he entered the spare room. It still had the old, dingy wallpaper, and for daylight it still depended on the two corner windows. It had been in a state of limbo ever since Amelia died. The sock monkey and the teddy bear and the yellow chick still waited expectantly.

"This is no way to deal with it," Dean said.

"I know." I wanted to talk, but I didn't know what to say. I just lay there, looking up at Dean standing by the door in his underwear, his hair sticking up comically on top of his head.

"You look like Alfalfa."

He reached up, feeling for the cowlick, tugging back on it. "Christ, do I not want to go to work," he said, looking up at the ceiling and heaving a sigh.

He went into the bathroom and started the shower, and I got up and went into the bathroom too and leaned on the sink with my left hand, staring at the shower curtain.

Somehow the hot, steamy air—and Dean's invisibility behind the curtain—made talking easier. My voice was pleading. "Some people think about their lives, the way they want to arrange things—their finances, their careers, their interests—and they decide that kids just aren't for them. That's okay. But to remain child-

less because you're just plain afraid of being hurt—
that's not a good reason. You don't really want to run
your life that way, do you?''

For a moment Dean said nothing. All I could hear
were my own thoughts and the rushing water. I wondered if I'd said the right thing.

But then he pushed the curtain aside and looked at
me. "You're right," he said, "I do want a child, I really
do."

The adoption agencies Dean and I had visited together in November were both local agencies devoted
to international adoption. I had learned about one of
them from a friend and the other from the Open Door
Society, an organization providing information and fel-
lowship for adoptive parents and would-be parents
and their children. At each agency, Dean and I met
privately with the director, explaining honestly that we
hadn't yet decided to adopt and were fearful of disappointment. The intimate atmosphere of these agencies
contrasted with the approach of the agency I had visited on my own, where the director, instead of meeting
couples individually, lectured to them in a large group.
There I had spent four hours taking notes on international adoption and observing the roomful of unhappy-
looking women and men. "Thank God Dean isn't here,"
I kept saying to myself. Looking around at the others, I
was convinced that we couldn't possibly all succeed in
our search.

But at the two private meetings, Dean and I were
told we could succeed. And we were made to feel that
we were just the sort of couple these agencies were
looking for. We needed this encouragement desperately, and I'm certain it helped Dean, weeks later, find
the courage to push his fears aside.

Ironically, both directors suggested we try looking
elsewhere. At domestic programs. Because we were

still emotionally spent, and because our medical problems had been so serious, they felt we should make domestic adoption our first choice. There would likely be more medical information available and thus fewer medical uncertainties. And we would escape the often lengthy waiting period between "assignment" of a child and arrival that makes the international process so grueling. "No," we heard, "it's not impossible to adopt an infant domestically."

But my investigations, in the weeks that followed, did not turn up many programs that Dean and I instinctively liked and felt we could count on to give us a child within the next year or two. In some ways, we limited our own options: we weren't interested in open adoption, where identities of all parties are shared; and we were afraid of so-called identified adoption, where a couple waits to receive the child of one particular woman's pregnancy rather than waiting for a placement from a pool of expectant women. We knew there would be risks in any adoption, but we didn't want to place our hopes in one woman; for us, if she lost her pregnancy or changed her mind, it would be too much like another stillbirth.

By mid-December, when Dean and I decided to adopt, we had crossed each of the domestic agencies off our list. Except one. There was one program we had a feeling about—that it wouldn't let us down, wouldn't put unnecessary obstacles in our path, wouldn't be insensitive to what we had been through. We just had this feeling, both of us. It had become in our minds *the* domestic program.

It was a program in Pennsylvania placing newborn babies, and it was the only program we had heard of that linked acceptance to an assurance that there would be a child. Though we had never visited the agency, never spoken to the people running it, we knew it worked. We had seen the evidence with our own eyes: two healthy little girls—the daughter of an old high school friend of mine, and, by coincidence, the daughter our doctor's friends had adopted.

My friend's little girl had been only ten days old when my friend and her husband had gone to Pennsylvania to receive her. And our doctor's friends had first held their little girl three days after her birth.

A newborn baby after all!

It was difficult not to get our hopes up; but my friend, and our doctor's friends, warned us that our chances of getting accepted were poor. The agency received over 5000 applications a year and accepted only about 125 couples, few of whom were from out of state.

"We shouldn't get too pumped up about this," Dean said, even as we began composing a letter.

It took us two weeks to write our letter, to find the right words to explain what we had been through—to present the facts of our story and to ask for something in return for our suffering. It exhausted us, and it made us feel terribly vulnerable. "Please," we wrote in our letter, "if you possibly can, help us."

Just a few days before we finished, Dean came home from work with strange news. Another lawyer in his law firm had just been accepted into the agency we were writing to.

A wave of anxiety went through me when I heard that. It meant the agency was definitely accepting couples from Massachusetts. But how many? Were we just in time? Or were we too late?

"Who are these people? How did they know about the agency?"

"From friends, I think. More or less the way we heard about it. Tom's a good guy. You'd like him."

"How about his wife? What's she like? What kinds of problems have they had?"

"I've met her once or twice. She seems nice. She can't get pregnant for some reason. I don't know the story. They've spent a fortune trying in vitro fertilization, going back and forth to some program in Virginia; every time they go, she has to have surgery. They were just down there recently and it didn't work out. Tom's depressed."

"I don't know what to feel. I should be happy for them for getting accepted, but all I keep thinking is, have they taken our spot?"

"That's ridiculous. It doesn't work that way."

On Saturday, January 18, we put the letter in the mail. "If they turn us down," Dean said, "there are other agencies, remember that."

"Maybe our luck will change. Maybe this time it will work the other way."

"Maybe so."

Monday was Martin Luther King Day, a federal holiday. No mail delivery. But on Tuesday I couldn't stop wondering whether our letter had been received.

Tuesday evening the phone rang, and something inside me, a little flare of optimism, made me think, what if? what if? Dean and I were watching television. I remember going into the kitchen to answer the phone.

It was the founder of the adoption agency. He had a soothing voice (sexy, I remember thinking afterwards, the way a man's voice is when it's protective, loving). "You're going to be a parent," he said, "you're going to be a parent. You can relax now, Marion. It's okay, you can relax."

And something in me—something clenched tight— finally did relax, begin to open, to breathe. My sleep was different that night; and the next morning, my waking. I *would* become a parent—I believed that now. It would take a while (probably by next Easter, he had said, a little more than a year), but it would happen.

"I feel like God called us last night," I said to Dean in the morning.

He laughed. "That wasn't God?"

A few days later, Dean and I went to a restaurant for dinner and I smiled back when the little boy in the booth behind Dean looked over and grinned at me. My smile was tentative; the little boy may not have even noticed it. But I felt it. An odd feeling, like using a limb that's been motionless for a long time.

"Do you think it's easier to die," I asked Dean, "if you've brought life into the world? You know, flesh of my flesh. . . ."

I was thinking of a dream I had had: I'm standing in the bathroom, an umbilical cord is hanging outside my swollen belly. The cord is thin and twisted and looks as though it may break off. I'm scared. I can't remember from prior pregnancies whether this is how the cord should look. I'm struggling to remember, frightened because I can't, and I call my mother into the bathroom, thinking she'll know, she'll tell me. Suddenly Death is standing in the hall. Its face is white, like a Kabuki actor's, expressionless, evil. I can't take my eyes off the face to look at the body, so I only sense the body. I have an impression of rich decoration, gold thread and ornaments, an elaborate arrangement of black hair piled up, shaped like a headdress. Is the figure male? The hair seems almost womanish. The figure is both sexes, but Death, definitely Death. I wake up just as I'm telling my mother to look, look.

"No," Dean said, "I don't think being a parent biologically makes it easier to die."

"But there's a kind of immortality in bearing a child, don't you think? I had this dream where I wanted my mother to save my baby; otherwise we would all die—not just the baby, but me and my mother too. I woke up blaming my mother. Because she couldn't help."

"Your question is confusing. Is it continuity you're thinking of? Generations? What if you have a child biologically and your kid gets hit by a truck? I keep telling you, there are no guarantees. You take what you get."

I was curled up on the couch in our living room. Feeling guilty. About my dream. About my constant doubting. Here I was, planning to adopt a child, and still thinking about pregnancy.

Dean paced slowly back and forth in front of me. For a while he stopped talking, his eyes almost closed in concentration, his thumb and forefinger drawing out the ends of his mustache as he paced. I liked watching him: walking towards me the length of the couch, taking a sip of bourbon from the glass on the mantle, then pivoting away from me, his back bent in thought. It was several minutes before he spoke again. "If you have an adopted child and that child has a child, do you doubt how much you'll love your grandchild? Do you think you'll be worrying about genes? Does it ever occur to you that you might be happier, more in love with your grandchild, because you've overcome so much to get there?"

"You really don't care about blood ties, do you?"

"No, I guess not, not the way you mean. Maybe it's because I never had aunts and uncles and cousins around when I was a kid. They were all out in Missouri. I don't know, maybe it's because the two kids next door were adopted. I never noticed their parents acting any different from mine."

Dean stopped pacing and stood by the couch and I reached up and hooked my fingers into his belt and pulled him closer.

"You talk as though there are categories of relationships," he said. "There aren't, there are only relationships. Look at you and me, you're closer to me than you are to anyone else. What has that got to do with blood?"

"But what about the love I felt when I was pregnant, that incredible connection? I miss that."

"I know you do." Dean was kneeling on the floor now, leaning over me, smoothing my hair. "But you'll love your child all the same. Don't confuse the high of being pregnant with the ability to love a child."

"Maybe you're right, maybe that's what I'm doing."
"Marion, you'll see—your child will show you."

"Did you feel angry when you began to realize how much would be demanded of you—the forms you would have to fill out, the medical reports, the meetings, the interviews?"

"Don't forget the FBI fingerprints," one of the men said. Everyone laughed.

Dean and I were at a preadoption meeting with six other couples, all of us seated around a table in a small windowless room at the adoption agency in Philadelphia. The agency's social worker stood at the head of the table asking us questions, encouraging us to talk. Her royal blue dress, the knitted fabric pulled tight over her hips and bust, was brighter than anything else in the room. She looked bold; cheerfully confident. It was October and our third trip to Philadelphia.

"I felt angry," Dean said. "Resentful. I mean, it seemed like all anyone else had to do to have a kid was screw, but we had to prove ourselves, even after what we'd already been through."

"I felt angry, too," one of the women said. She spoke softly, nervously. "You start to think, when will it end? Will I pass all the tests? Will I say something wrong?"

"I felt the same way," said Carla, Tom's wife, "but you know, I also think there's something good about all the requirements. I feel chosen. Anyone can have a child the other way."

"Anyone but us," Dean quipped, waving his hand in an arc that indicated all of the couples at the table.

Carla laughed. She had a bubbling laugh; hearty, unconstrained, with no sharp edges; it contrasted with her straight-backed posture, her formal clothes, her aura of refinement.

When Dean had introduced me to Carla and Tom on

our first train trip to Philadelphia in August, I had liked them instantly. They were fun to be with—talkative, playful, conspiratorial. And they seemed as eager for our friendship as we were for theirs. Between the four of us, there was an immediate intimacy, and our train trips together accelerated the normal pace of friendship. We spent hours discussing our families, our fears about adoption, our medical histories, our tentative new hopes. A mantle of mutual understanding, tact and encouragement drew us together, much as if the four of us had pulled one great blanket around our shoulders.

The adoption agency had accepted fifty-seven couples to attend meetings that fall, only seven of them from Massachusetts: the seven seated in that small room. As out-of-staters, expatriates of a sort, we established an animated camaraderie before the start of the meeting, trading travel and hotel stories, making plans to get together back home, coaching each other on how to handle the red tape at the Massachusetts end. We would be meeting together all day—from ten in the morning until late in the afternoon, and this would be our first and last small-group meeting; the August and September meetings had been held in a large lecture room with all fifty-seven couples present; the November meeting, the last meeting we were required to attend, would return to the lecture format.

As the social worker began asking questions, directing the conversation, I was censoring my comments carefully. I felt myself under scrutiny, much more than at the larger meetings, and in spite of the stated purpose of this meeting—to teach us about the special concerns of adoptive parents and their children, and to help the social worker get to know us—I persisted in thinking of the meeting as a test that each of us had to pass. Carla and Tom had told me they felt the same way.

"Has anyone ever failed to be approved?" someone asked.

"It happens," the social worker said. "But it's usually more a matter of the couple removing themselves from the process. Generally people recognize problems themselves."

"But what would be some of the reasons for rejecting a couple?"

"You tell me."

"Alcoholism?" someone offered. The social worker began a list on the blackboard.

"Financial instability?"

"Mental problems?"

"What about if you're just not ready yet?" asked Kim, the woman sitting next to Tom. "What if you haven't reached what I call your breaking point?" She was short, heavyset, with bobbed dirty-blond hair and large, impatient eyes; and she was demonstrative, garrulous, her hands clasping and separating as she spoke, her eyes staring around the table. Her husband, Bill, seated to her right, was thin and quiet. "I know exactly when I reached my breaking point. It was after my last operation. I just knew I couldn't keep trying, I just couldn't keep running my life that way."

I liked hearing her story. I didn't mind her using up time to tell it. I knew what she meant about breaking points, and I liked hearing it from someone else. I kept nodding at her, staring back at her as if to say, "Go on, go on."

"Maybe it's different for some of you," she said, "but I know I couldn't focus on adoption and my own infertility at the same time. I couldn't try to adopt until I stopped running from doctor to doctor."

"But what about the hurt?" the social worker asked.

"What do you mean?"

"Well, the hurt, the disappointment—you wanted a pregnancy so much. What do you do with the hurt?"

"I don't . . ." Kim looked down at the table. "I'm not sure." She could hardly speak. I thought she might cry.

The social worker looked questioningly around the table. No one spoke. Finally, the social worker sat down and leaned towards Kim.

"You'll always have that hurt," she said. "Take it and wrap it up and set it aside and accept the fact that it's yours. You don't need to throw it away. You can't. Sometimes you'll take it up for a moment and have a good cry. Don't feel guilty. Even when you have your child, don't feel guilty. It doesn't mean you don't love your child. That's something separate."

Carla was sitting next to me, and I reached for her hand. I knew before she even turned to look at me that her eyes would be filled with tears like mine.

It was around three-thirty in the afternoon when the phone rang in the room where we were meeting. "You have a call, Bill," the social worker said. Kim's husband took the phone while the rest of us joked about some people just being *too* indispensable to their employers. But then someone was saying, "Shhh, shhh," and we were all staring at Bill; the blood had drained from his face, and he was pressing the receiver hard against his ear, motioning the rest of us to be quiet.

"What is it, what is it?" Kim asked, shaking him by the shoulder. He motioned her to lean toward him and he whispered something in her ear.

I think we all understood at that moment—felt it, rather than heard it; knew it before it was said: there was a child waiting for them. The agency director was calling with the news.

Kim rose to her feet, her arms outstretched, like a sleepwalker's, and she stood there, grabbing for support in the air, wailing hysterically, laughing, sobbing, gasping for breath.

I felt no jealousy for once, none at all. Only joy for them. I was crying with joy for them. And I was laughing, too.

Dean put his arm around me. I leaned forward for a

moment, resting my head on the table, listening to Kim's wailing: "A boy . . . a boy . . . I have a boy!" I wanted to fix that sound in my mind. That mixture of pain and joy and love and unbearable relief.

That night I dreamed that Dean and I had received our call. I had been out somewhere, and the agency director had reached Dean at his office. We had traveled to the agency, and now we were walking toward the door to the room that held our child. I hadn't yet asked Dean the child's sex, but just in front of the closed door I stopped and grabbed his arm, tugging at him. He stood still and looked at me.

"Tell me," I asked, "what did they give us? What is it?"

"Open the door, open the door and see."

I gripped his arm so hard I could feel my clenched fist aching through my dream. He took my hand and held it, and I had a vague sense of Dean, in bed, lying beside me. "Are you all right? You're dreaming. Are you all right?"

In my dream I stared into Dean's eyes—those gentle eyes, not quite gray, not quite blue—and slowly, slowly, with my free hand I reached for the door.

EPILOGUE

In 1987, Dean and I brought our baby home—a little girl.